OUR
IDENTITY

DEFINED BY GOD, NOT BY SIN

DR. HENRY W. WRIGHT

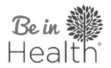

4178 Crest Highway

Thomaston, Georgia 30286

www.beinhealth.com

ISBN 978-1-61184-163-3

Copyright Notice

TABLE OF CONTENTS

DISCLAIMER

We do not seek to be in conflict with any medical or psychiatric practices, or any church or its religious doctrines, beliefs, or practices. We are not part of medicine or psychology; we are working to make them more effective, believing that many human problems are fundamentally spiritual, with associated physiological and psychological manifestations. This information is intended for your general knowledge only, to give insight into disease, its problems, and possible solutions. It is not a substitute for medical advice or treatment from specific medical conditions or disorders. We do not diagnose or treat disease. You should seek prompt medical care for any specific health issues. Treatment modalities around your specific health issues are between you and your physician. We are not responsible for a person's disease or their healing. We are administering the Scriptures and what they say about this subject, along with what the medical and scientific communities have observed in line with this insight. There is no guarantee any person will be healed or any disease prevented. The fruits of this teaching will come forth out of the application of the principles and the relationship between each person and God. Be in Health® is patterned after 2 Corinthians 5:18-20, 1 Corinthians 12, Ephesians 4, and Mark 16:15-20.

Foreword

My husband, Dr. Henry Wright, was in ministry for over 30 years and was known for his teachings that brought healing to many people spiritually, emotionally, and physically. He was passionate about helping Believers learn to be overcomers. And he loved teaching foundational Biblical principles in a way that anyone could understand.

The teaching on *Our Identity* was developed many years ago and was one of Henry's most important messages. He wanted everyone to know who they are in God because he believed that finding our identity was paramount to being an overcomer. Without understanding our identity, we don't know who we are fighting or what the battleground is.

He wanted people to know who they are and where they came from, so they would know where they are going. When people see the big picture, they begin to understand that they truly belong to God. Situations in our lives come and go, but a sense of belonging and identity can only come from God.

Henry's desire was to release this teaching years ago; however, God's timing is always perfect! A huge thanks to the team who worked on this book—a special thanks to Scott Iwahashi for his intense perseverance for bringing Henry's voice to the present. And thanks to God for the understanding He has entrusted us with.

Now is the time to unearth the treasure of who we are in Him.

- Pastor Donna Wright, Co-Founder of Be in Health®

Chapter 1: The Journey of Sanctification

OLD THINGS ARE PASSED AWAY

In Christianity, what we are taught to believe about our identity as a child of God often does not match the reality of our lives. Much of what we are told describes a hypothetical existence. Over the years, many believers have come to me for ministry. If becoming a believer meant all our problems disappeared, why do people still come to me for help? If the hypothetic idea was true that our old man was completely gone when we were born again, there would be no need for ministry.

I have had to grapple with the subject of what happens to us spiritually when we become born again. The concept in Christianity is that when we are born again, "old things are passed away; behold, all things are become new" — therefore, there is no more evil in our lives. However, in ministry, I bumped into a rude awakening. Many Christians I ministered to were more evil than the world. I am not trying to denigrate the Church; I am being very honest. Discovering that born-again Christians had as much evil in them as unregenerated humans was a staggering revelation.

This observation led me to an investigation into the New Testament and some word studies in the Greek language to understand this phenomenon.

I realized that when we became born again, our spirits had become alive to God in spite of the devil. After becoming born again, we are still on a journey to overcome Satan's kingdom. And from this starting point, we enter into something called sanctification. Why would we need to be sanctified if there was no more evil in us when we became born again? If I did not believe that a Christian could have evil, then nobody would get well through this church and ministry.

Now, I want to address a question—someone might ask what died when they were born again. This question would be in reference to 2 Corinthians 5:17.

> *Therefore if any man be in Christ, he is a new creature: old things are passed away; behold, all things are become new. 2 Corinthians 5:17 KJV*

What died or passed away? Let us address this passage by unfolding its meaning. We are saved by faith, are we not? We still are to this day. The object of our belief has not come to pass. We are much the same as every other person walking on this planet, except our spirits have come alive to God. Because the Holy Spirit has come to live with us, we are now able to overcome evil. According to Scripture, they overcame Satan by the blood of the Lamb and by the word of their testimony.

> *And they overcame him by the blood of the Lamb, and by the word of their testimony; and they loved not their*

lives unto the death. Revelation 12:11 KJV

And the great miracle of this journey is that by faith, as a work of the Holy Spirit and the Word of God, we are able to be holy as He is holy, and we can subdue evil and be changed. So what did die? To be honest, nothing. Perhaps we should ask instead: what came alive when we were born again? The answer is our spirit came alive to God. Satan is still on the earth, but we have the ability to resist him and his kingdom.

SPIRITUAL WORLD REALITY

Now, we come to two dimensions essential to our health and healing. The first dimension is sanctification, and the second is the removal of Satan's influence over our lives. I have had to address this subject with people in order to get them well. In my teachings on the subject of Spirit World Realities, I go into depth defining Satan's kingdom according to Scripture. I address what sin is, where it comes from, where it is today, and what it is doing. In discussing Spirit World Realities, I unfold something called the second heaven. It is my position that the first heaven is the physical dimension of creation, where we interact with the world around us with our five physical senses. In the future, the first heaven and earth will pass away when the New Heaven and New Earth are established.

And I saw a new heaven and a new earth: for the first heaven and the first

earth were passed away; and there was
no more sea. Revelation 21:1 KJV

The third heaven is where Father God lives.
We do not see the third heaven with our physical
eyes, but it is a spiritual dimension described by the
Scriptures.

I knew a man in Christ above fourteen
years ago, (whether in the body, I
cannot tell; or whether out of the body, I
cannot tell: God knoweth;) such an one
caught up to the third heaven. 2
Corinthians 12:2 KJV

While it is not explicitly stated in Scripture, it is
my position that the second heaven is referred to as
the "dry place." It is not the third heaven where God
lives, nor is it part of the first heaven as part of our
physical creation; therefore, by inference, I have
interpreted the "dry place" to be the second heaven.
When evil spirits are cast out of humans, they go to
the "dry place," a place of torment to them because
they can no longer manifest evil through our lives.

When the unclean spirit is gone out of a
man, he walketh through dry places,
seeking rest, and findeth none. Matthew
12:43 KJV

BODY, SOUL, SPIRIT

Two dimensions are important to our life and
freedom. In order to remove Satan's kingdom, we

must understand it, but we also need to understand how Father God designed humans. To understand sanctification, we need to examine the three components of every human. According to Scripture, we are a spirit, we have a soul, and we live in a body. We are a triune being.

> *And the very God of peace sanctify you wholly; and I pray God your whole spirit and soul and body be preserved blameless unto the coming of our Lord Jesus Christ. 1 Thessalonians 5:23 KJV*

To understand this subject, it is important to differentiate our spirit from our soul. Our spirit is not a physical part of our creation. The best we can gather from Scripture is that our spirit resides around our belly. For this reason, when we are tempted by sin, we do not feel it in our mind/soul but around our belly. When we are angry, we feel a "high octane ping" on the inside, and when we feel afraid, we may feel nervousness and uneasiness in our gut.

> *He that believeth on me, as the scripture hath said, out of his belly shall flow rivers of living water. John 7:38 KJV*

> *The spirit of man is the candle of the LORD, searching all the inward parts of the belly. Proverbs 20:27 KJV*

It is my position that the soul is our mind, where we think and reason. So when we are being sanctified, what part of us is being sanctified? If we are born again, our soul is the part of us being sanctified. Once an evil spirit is cast out of us, it is our soul that is being renewed according to the Word of God. Paul dealt with this issue. He addressed this subject in 2 Corinthians 7:1.

LET US CLEANSE OURSELVES

Before going there, I want to reiterate what I said previously: when we became born again, what died? Well, nothing. It is what came alive in us. We came alive to the reality that we are to establish the Kingdom of God in the midst of the kingdom of evil. That is what changed and continues to change by our obedience.

Now, let us go back to 2 Corinthians 7:1.

Having therefore these promises, dearly beloved, let us cleanse ourselves from all filthiness of the flesh and spirit, perfecting holiness in the fear of God.
2 Corinthians 7:1 KJV

We read: "Having therefore these promises, dearly beloved." This is being addressed to Christians. "Let us cleanse ourselves from all filthiness of the flesh and spirit, perfecting holiness in the fear of God."

Is this before conversion or after conversion? It is AFTER conversion. Now, what makes it possible is that our spirit comes alive to God after we become born again. Before we were born again, what was our relationship to God? We were dead to God in our trespasses and sins. However, we may have had some serious spiritual issues when we were born again. When we became born again, we may have had an evil spirit in us — we may even have had a legion. I have found Christians with legions of evil spirits in them.

I know some people teach that Christians cannot have evil spirits; however, they do not have a leg to stand on doctrinally. There is not one Scripture that they have to prove that position. So I do not debate the question of whether or not a Christian can have an evil spirit. If I am asked this question, I ask my own in response: "Can an evil spirit have a Christian?" In other words, are evil spirits pulling our strings through temptation and thoughts meant to control our actions? By this standard, they can, and they have.

I have cast out legions from Christians. During New Testament Biblical times, a legion consisted of thousands of soldiers. I ministered to one person that had three legions. It called itself by name; it identified itself, and I cast out three legions. So I have found evil spirits in Christians. These were born-again Christians.

THE PROCESS OF BEING TRANSFORMED

How are we born again? We accept the promises of God, by faith. Are we going to heaven? Are we there yet? How do we know we are going to get there in the future? By faith. Has the object of our faith, in regard to our salvation, come to pass yet? Not yet. We are going to have to wait and see how this thing turns out after we die. In the meantime, the Holy Spirit is here working with us. We are being changed as we follow Father God. Remember the Scripture: "from glory to glory" we are being changed.

> *But we all, with open face beholding as in a glass the glory of the Lord, are changed into the same image from glory to glory, even as by the Spirit of the Lord. 2 Corinthians 3:18 KJV*

If we are born again, why would we need to be changed "from glory to glory"? If our spiritual journey was totally finished when we were born again, why would we need to be changed "from glory to glory" into His image? Because our journey has not finished. Have we ever noticed that when a person is born again, they often struggle with the same evil they had before they became born again?

The problem is that we struggle with understanding what was supposed to have passed away when we were born again. As a reminder, what passed away? Nothing passed away; it is what came alive. However, what if we are on the journey of something passing away? See, we have present progressive tense here (an ongoing, current action). We find in Scripture a critical concept—it is called present progressive. What is faith? Present progressive. We are in the process of being transformed. Now, we are told to leave those things that are behind and press on to the mark of the high calling of God in Christ Jesus.

> *Therefore if any man be in Christ, he is a new creature: old things are passed away; behold, all things are become new. 2 Corinthians 5:17 KJV*

> *I press toward the mark for the prize of the high calling of God in Christ Jesus. Philippians 3:14 KJV*

In Revelation it says, "he that overcometh shall inherit all things."

> *He that overcometh shall inherit all things; and I will be his God, and he shall be my son. Revelation 21:7 KJV*

Then what are we overcoming? We might say we are overcoming the devil, but it is important to understand that we are not overcoming Satan himself. The devil is not omnipresent. He is not omniscient. We know from Scripture that only God is omniscient or all-knowing. Only God is omnipresent or present everywhere at once. If anyone wants to see this for themselves, refer to Job 1. The following is my interpretation of their interaction. When the sons of God came to present themselves before the Lord,

Satan came with them. And the Lord said to Satan, "What have you been up to?" Satan replied that he was walking to and fro, up and down the earth. If the devil were everywhere at one time, he would not need to travel from place to place.

> *⁶Now there was a day when the sons of God came to present themselves before the LORD, and Satan came also among them. ⁷And the LORD said unto Satan, Whence comest thou? Then Satan answered the LORD, and said, From going to and fro in the earth, and from walking up and down in it. Job 1:6-7 KJV*

THE SANCTIFICATION OF OUR SPIRIT

Now, part of the revelation and understanding needed for our freedom and health relates to what was lost at the fall of Adam and Eve in the Garden of Eden. We need to define what it means to say that "sin came into the world." Mankind became sinful as a result of the fall. However, we cannot just inspect the evil that came into creation to gain our freedom.

> *Wherefore, as by one man sin entered into the world, and death by sin; and so death passed upon all men, for that all have sinned: Romans 5:12 KJV*

It is essential to have a revelation of what this planet was supposed to be like according to Father God's plan. When we have a revelation of what the nature of man should have been — when we have a revelation of what the work of sanctification means — then we can turn away from the works of evil and toward the works of righteousness. Now, it is important to understand sanctification is not a work of the flesh. We do not become sanctified on our own. It is by the work of the Holy Spirit that we are sanctified.

But, in order to move forward, I want to take the contrary position. If one were to argue that our spirit is already entirely sanctified before God, why would we need to overcome? And why would Paul say we are to cleanse ourselves from all filthiness of the flesh and spirit?

> *Having therefore these promises, dearly beloved, let us cleanse ourselves from all filthiness of the flesh and spirit, perfecting holiness in the fear of God. 2 Corinthians 7:1 KJV*

Paul dealt with this subject clearly in Romans 7. Romans 7 cuts through this argument for me in helping people to overcome sin in their lives. Paul had been an apostle for 20-plus years when he wrote Romans, and he was dealing with a very real and present issue. Before we look at his words, it is important to understand that the only difference separating me from an unsaved person is my obedience to God. See, there are disobedient spirits, and there are obedient spirits. Satan was a disobedient spirit. One-third of all angels were disobedient spirits. All the beings that fell with Lucifer and the third of the angels in the world before Adam were disobedient spirits. All of mankind today who are separated from God are disobedient spirits.

At the core, I am a spirit. How do I know I am a spirit? Because the Word of God says that I am a spirit. The Word of God says God is the Father of all spirits.

> *Furthermore we have had fathers of our flesh which corrected us, and we gave them reverence: shall we not much rather be in subjection unto the Father of spirits, and live? Hebrews 12:9 KJV*

Scriptures also say that I am a son of God.

> *He that overcometh shall inherit all things; and I will be his God, and he shall be my son. Revelation 21:7 KJV*

So if God is the Father of all spirits and I am also a son of God, I am a spirit first. If God is my Father, I must be a spirit with a soul who lives in a body. First Thessalonians 5:23 is a pivotal connection point in this discussion to prove our three-dimensional makeup as humans. This leads back to my main point of addressing our identity.

First Thessalonians 5:23 begins by saying, "the very God of peace sanctify you." However, the next word is not what we would expect—it says *wholly*. It is not spelled h-o-l-y; it is spelled w-h-o-l-l-y. This is essential to our discussion because *wholly* means fully in spirit, soul, and body. This is the process of sanctification, and it includes spirit, soul, and body. May the God of peace sanctify us wholly: w-h-o-l-l-y, in spirit, soul, and body.

> *And the very God of peace sanctify you wholly; and I pray God your whole spirit and soul and body be preserved blameless unto the coming of our Lord Jesus Christ. 1 Thessalonians 5:23 KJV*

So here is a three-dimensional description of our existence. We are a spirit, have a soul, and live in a body.

WE DO NOT COHABITATE WITH THE ENEMY

Hebrews 4:12 says the Word of God is quick and powerful, sharper than a two-edged sword, able to penetrate even to the joint and marrow, is a discerner of the thoughts and intents of the heart, and is able to separate the soul from the spirit.

> *For the word of God is quick, and powerful, and sharper than any twoedged sword, piercing even to the dividing asunder of soul and spirit, and of the joints and marrow, and is a discerner of the thoughts and intents of the heart. Hebrews 4:12 KJV*

So the soul and the spirit are uniquely separate and different. Psychology has done us a great disservice because Carl Jung and Jungian psychology teaches a dualistic compartment of the soul and denies the existence of the human spirit. In fact, in Jungian psychology, there is the soul and another compartment known as the collective subconscious. According to Jung, the collective subconscious is where the archetypes and dark shadows of our psyche are located.

However, when we study the historical writings of Carl Jung, he decided to commit a sleight of hand change of terminology. Before he used psychological terminology, he acknowledged that archetypes and dark shadows were evil spirits. However, he changed the name from evil spirits to archetypes and dark shadows because secular society and science would not accept references to spirits. He tapped into what he called the ancestral archetypes of the darkness of our generations. Well, what are they? As Christians, we know them to be evil spirits.

Years ago, I created a pamphlet, and I subtly inserted something to see who would read it. I wanted to see who would read and pay attention to the connection I had drawn. I was testing the waters and bridging together concepts. The pamphlet said "spirits of infirmity and spirits of insanity: archetypes and dark shadows revealed." That was all it said. It was just a two-line statement, and as our literature was going across America, I waited for somebody to put two and two together. Yes, that is exactly what I intended.

Eventually, we had a couple of psychotherapists come to visit from north of Atlanta. They were a very nice couple who were both psychotherapists. They were Christians who had accepted our teachings and had been applying the principles to their practice. Both of them told me they were achieving success in their practice because they were identifying the archetypes and dark shadows as evil spirits. As believers, they cast them out. In most of psychotherapy, they do not cast out evil spirits. In psychotherapy, they generally teach us how to live with our evil. Psychotherapy teaches us how to identify our evil and come into a place of cohabitation with it. We are told that we will be able to coexist with our problem and have a better life. We do not have freedom, but we have a measure of relief because we are less tormented by the evil spirits that we adopted as part of our personalities.

On the other hand, the Bible says something different about Jesus, our Lord. It says that whom the Son sets free is free indeed. Therefore, I do not teach cohabitation with an enemy.

If the Son therefore shall make you free, ye shall be free indeed. John 8:36 KJV

I teach the elimination of the enemy for freedom because that is what I see in Scripture. I am not interested in practicing the principles of psychotherapy. However, I have studied psychotherapy and the principles of Jungian psychology. Jungian psychology teaches the dualistic compartment of the soul. There is no such thing. In fact, I am not alone in this conclusion. Many years ago, I heard Charles Capps' teaching on the very same topic of what psychology calls the collective subconscious. His conclusion was the fact that it describes the spirit of man found in Scripture. I agree with this position, and I have agreed with it for a long time. So, from a Scriptural standpoint, that is what I see. It is vital to our discussion to understand that we do not cohabit with evil spirits but cast them out. Without casting out evil spirits, we do not have freedom.

WORK OUT OUR SALVATION

Moving on, we must address the two parts of a human that need to be spiritually cleansed. One is the flesh, and the other one is the spirit. What is the flesh, and what is the spirit? Many people say Paul's thorn in the flesh was a disease because they think the word *flesh* refers to our human body. When we look up the word *flesh* and evaluate it in the Biblical context, we find it has nothing to do with our human body.

In Romans 7, I have found the word *flesh* refers to the "old nature" otherwise known as the sin nature. The old nature can be dualistic because we do not have the discernment to separate ourselves from evil spirits manifesting in our lives without the Spirit of God. Sometimes we seem more sane, and other times we manifest evil — and we have no idea what is coming out of us. It is almost as if we had a split personality.

This teaching does not cover the soul in depth because that would require a specific examination on its own. Some have wanted me to teach on the soul for a while, but they do not understand how long it would take me. I take the time to answer questions because I want to be able to develop a topic. I do not want to give someone a flippant answer because thoughtful answers require exploring what Father God has said in His Word. In order for us to be fully persuaded from the Word of God, we need to carefully examine what it has said.

In Christendom, especially in some charismatic circles, there is a great gap between promises and reality. Everything is taught in terms of promises. Well, is that not what faith is? The problem is not found in the promises of God. However, the promises have to do with the completeness of our metamorphosis, and one day we will all be complete. But when? In heaven? Does that mean we have to wait to get to heaven for the metamorphosis to begin? No, we are working out our own salvation daily with fear and trembling.

> *Wherefore, my beloved, as ye have always obeyed, not as in my presence only, but now much more in my absence, work out your own salvation with fear and trembling. Philippians 2:12 KJV*

Many people who become born again fall into the trap of eternal security. These concepts suggest that we do not have to worry about sanctification once we are born again. And to be honest, many of those denominations do not teach sanctification. If they do, it is from the standpoint of legalism. They define rules and regulations for Christians that extend well beyond the Bible. Their focus is on curbing evil behavior and what they define as right and wrong. Oftentimes, they threaten their people and use fear as a means to scare them away from doing evil.

The point of sanctification is not to be changed because I am being forced into it. I am not allowing the Holy Spirit to change me because I am afraid the alternative is hell. I am not doing it because I am afraid of God. I want to be like my Father. I want my nature to be transformed because I want to be exactly what He created me to be — not in order to conform to a religious image made up by someone else. I believe the purpose of ministry is to strip away the expectations of others, including a husband, wife, parents, or friends, and present a person back to Father God. I want to let them be exactly what He wanted them to be from the foundation of the world. This requires that I confront these expectations with the Word of God. If they have been told they are unlovable by humans, and Scripture says the opposite — they must decide whom to believe. Their decision requires repenting to Father God for believing these lies and returning to what He has said about them. That is how I think. I, myself, am in the process of walking in what He planned for me from the foundation of the world according to the Scriptures of the Bible.

DO NOT BELIEVE THE LIES

When I first came to the Lord, I was a prodigal. I came to the Lord at 38 years of age after wandering for 13 or 14 years. I attended a large church of approximately 1,500 people when I was first born again. A known Prophet occasionally visited our church; he did not attend that church, but he knew the Pastor. He did not know me from a hole in the ground, and I did not know him either. During one Thursday night service with 1,000 people in attendance, right in the middle of praise and worship, he walked down to the front and whispered in the Pastor's ear. That service came to a grinding halt. He turned around and said, "God has just spoken to me, and I must do what He told me to do." And he said, "There's one person here that God has a word for." He turned around and looked through the whole congregation. He pointed with his finger, "You, come here." He was not smiling.

In this large service, everybody looked around to see who it was. I was wearing a little sports jacket. I did not have a beard; I just had a mustache. I assumed he was not looking at me. However, to make a long story short, he was interested in me. As soon as I realized it, I mentally began going through my sin list quickly. I checked my sin list because I did not want to be called out in a church service. No one wants to be called out of a service by a prophet for that reason. Either God is speaking to a person about His plans for them, or He is going to tell them to shape up or ship out by repenting for sin. Most people would be apprehensive, too, would they not? I walked down that long aisle and stood before him, and he prophesied over me in tongues. The Pastor interpreted, which authenticated it for me. If it had only been in English, then that probably would have been fine, but the prophecy in tongues by the Prophet with the Pastor's interpretation was a verification because of the level of discernment of both men. I considered that to be significant and still do.

I do not remember everything said that day, but I do remember part of it. The reason why I am addressing this subject is that we are addressing the topic of our identity. The key to addressing our identity is to expose our underlying insecurities. We have questions and concerns about this topic. Who are we? We usually do not want to answer that question too quickly because we are about 50-50; in other words, we feel as if we are half of the devil and half of God these days. And half of us is full of truth, and half is full of error. Half is full of righteousness, half is full of evil. If that were not the case, we would not need to be sanctified. We would be sinless just like the Lord, and there is not a person on the face of this earth who is sinless. There is not a person on the face of this earth who is not working out some sin issue in their life — or should be. If they claim they do not have to address any sin in their lives, they are a liar, and they are in denial.

Returning to the prophecy, there was a part I will always remember and never forget. It burns within me. I liken it to when the angel came to Mary about the Lord; she pondered these things in her heart.

But Mary kept all these things, and pondered them in her heart. Luke 2:19 KJV

Way back then, I was not yet in ministry. I was just a sheep sitting in the congregation. I had been back with the Lord maybe nine months, and I was just growing up in Him in learning and reading the Bible. However, in the midst of my journey as an unknown person to that Prophet, the Lord must have known me because I will never forget what he said as long as I live. It burns within me like a fire all the time. "You," God said, "You are mine. You belong to me. I have called you to do a work in your generation. Be all that I have called you to be, and do not listen to lies." That is all I remember, and that is enough for me.

Do we truly believe He has called us to be His sons and daughters? Will we listen to Satan's lies that tell us we have no value? I cannot make that decision for anyone. God has said it, but whether we repent, resist lies, and choose to believe Him or not is our choice. Do we believe we are fearfully and wonderfully made?

> [13]For thou hast possessed my reins: thou hast covered me in my mother's womb. [14]I will praise thee; for I am fearfully and wonderfully made: marvellous are thy works; and that my soul knoweth right well. Psalm 139:13-14 KJV

WHAT IS OUR IDENTITY?

For us to be what Father God has said we are, we must be willing to conform to His Word. Sanctification has to begin for vessels of honor to be perfected.

> [20]Nay but, O man, who art thou that repliest against God? Shall the thing formed say to him that formed it, Why hast thou made me thus? [21]Hath not the potter power over the clay, of the same lump to make one vessel unto honour, and another unto dishonour? Romans 9:20-21 KJV

Do we want to be a vessel of honor? Do we want to be a split personality–half representing the devil and half representing God? Do we want to be full of truth or full of divination? Do we want to be full of love or full of hate? Do we want to be full of forgiveness or full of bitterness? Do we want to be full of strife or full of peacemaking? Who do we want to be? Do we want to be somebody who builds up others or tears them down? Do we want to be somebody who edifies or somebody who does not? Who are we going to be?

So, what is our identity?

Chapter 2: The Law of Sin

THE TRUE MEASURE OF SPIRITUALITY

Our identity is to be an extension of the living God, and the living God is not evil. The living God is known by His character or nature. To understand ourselves, we must look at the characteristics of the living God. Before going forward, it is essential to understand that the "fruit of the Spirit" is the fruit of the Holy Spirit. The capital *S* Spirit manifests His character through humans who choose to follow Father God. These characteristics are known as the fruit of the Holy Spirit and reflect Father God's nature.

> *22But the fruit of the Spirit is love, joy, peace, longsuffering, gentleness, goodness, faith, 23Meekness, temperance: against such there is no law. Galatians 5:22-23 KJV*

The world, apart from God, behaves contrary to the Word of God. In this way, they follow what Jesus said to the Pharisees when He told them their father was the devil. Jesus was not slandering them or calling them names. He was pointing out the fact that their character and nature were reflective of Satan's kingdom.

> *Ye are of your father the devil, and the lusts of your father ye will do. He was a murderer from the beginning, and abode*

not in the truth, because there is no
truth in him. When he speaketh a lie, he
speaketh of his own: for he is a liar, and
the father of it. John 8:44 KJV

Therefore, the Scriptures instruct us so that we may follow Father God as His children. The Bible says, "A soft answer turneth away wrath."

A soft answer turneth away wrath: but
grievous words stir up anger. Proverbs
15:1 KJV

It also says, "Blessed are the merciful: for they shall obtain mercy."

Blessed are the merciful: for they shall
obtain mercy. Matthew 5:7 KJV

Many parts of the Church judge spirituality by whether a person can prophesy or their charismatic persona. I do not use such a measure. My test of the true spirituality of a person is how much more normal, in a good sense, they are. A truer barometer of spirituality is how normal a human being behaves rather than how much they prophesy. I see many evil people prophesy. It is not how many people they heal; I have seen evil people heal. When the Word of God is preached or practiced, Father God will meet people in their needs according to their faith. The danger is that many ministers believe they did it themselves when people are healed, or the Spirit of God uses them to speak. In fact, the Word says it—

there will be those who come before Him in that day and say they have cast out devils in His name, they have healed the sick in His name, and they have prophesied. And Jesus will say, "I never knew you: depart from Me."

> ²¹*Not every one that saith unto me, Lord, Lord, shall enter into the kingdom of heaven; but he that doeth the will of my Father which is in heaven. ²²Many will say to me in that day, Lord, Lord, have we not prophesied in thy name? and in thy name have cast out devils? and in thy name done many wonderful works? ²³And then will I profess unto them, I never knew you: depart from me, ye that work iniquity. Matthew 7:21-23 KJV*

What do we do with that Scripture? I am not impressed with people operating in the gifts of the Holy Spirit. It does not impress me in the slightest. If someone comes around operating in the gifts of the Spirit with a lot of hype and all that stuff, I am not impressed whatsoever. I am not impressed with people who prophesy and people who do miracles. I am interested in who they are as a person. I am interested in their heart. I am interested in finding out if I can "take them to the bank." By that, I mean to say that I want to know if I can trust my life with them. Are they trustworthy? Will they tell the truth and admit when they have failings and sins in their lives?

I am interested in a person's character. I am not interested in how high they can fly or their level of hype. I am interested in how close they can be to other humans and how much they love others. That is the true test. That is why I get a little nervous around the prophetic movements that have become popular because there does not seem to be a whole lot of teaching of sanctification going along with it. It is important not to lump everyone together, but there have been a lot of unsanctified people being exalted as "high flyers", but their lives are a tragedy. I am bothered when I do not see sanctification in conjunction with the works of God. It bothers me when I do not see sanctification tied to any movements.

WE MUST ADDRESS THE SPIRITUAL ISSUE

I hope this does not seem like a negative statement but rather a challenging one. We need to realize that we are to be working out our own salvation daily with fear and trembling.

> *Wherefore, my beloved, as ye have always obeyed, not as in my presence only, but now much more in my absence, work out your own salvation with fear and trembling. Philippians 2:12 KJV*

Everyone has something in their lives that does not line up with the Word of God. We all know it. With many types of disease, I can give at least a dozen spiritual issues wrong in a person's life that must be straightened out so that will lead to healing. Without going into a great deal of depth, we can see there are problems in our lives. We are able to address many diseases, and there are spiritual problems.

If not for these sin issues, we would not be struggling with many diseases. How can that be? Well, in Romans 7, Paul deals with this subject in verse 15. Verse 15 in the King James Version is a little difficult to understand on its own. With the help of verse 16, I will help us work through this subject of sin to give us the cause and the understanding of the battle over it in our lives. Paul develops this theme line by line in these Scriptures. As an important note, Paul is speaking as a born-again Christian who is on a journey. He is also an apostle to the Gentiles. It is my position that he is not speaking in the past tense when he talks about his journey with sin. Some people may suggest he was speaking hypothetically or in the past tense, but I believe he is being transparent about his present journey to overcome sin in his own life.

It states in verse 15 (my paraphrase), "For that which I do I allow not: for what I would (or what I would want to do), I do not do it. And those things that I hate, that is what I do."

> *For that which I do I allow not: for what I would, that do I not; but what I hate, that do I. Romans 7:15 KJV*

It goes on in Romans 7:16:

If then I do that which I would not, I
consent unto the law that it is good.
Romans 7:16 KJV

What law are we consenting to when we sin against God? It is the law of sin manifesting in our members, otherwise known as our body, when we speak or act in a way contrary to the Bible.

But I see another law in my members,
warring against the law of my mind,
and bringing me into captivity to the
law of sin which is in my members.
Romans 7:23 KJV

We do not want to serve sin, but when we follow after thoughts of temptation that contradict the Word of God, we are in bondage to the law of sin. Have any of us, as Christians, ever found ourselves doing something evil, hated it, and could not stop ourselves? Or are we just in denial about an issue? We need to stop denying the sin issues in our lives. There are some people in Christianity who live in extreme denial of their issues. If we are not careful, we can be drawn into certain sects of Christianity that propel us into a hyper range of "faith" where we are not allowed to be weak and have issues. They reason that if someone is weak, it is a sign of faithlessness, and they will ostracize others for it.

Rather than deal with the issues of life, people can go into a sort of hyper-faith where they do not admit their faults and problems. They are forced to make positive "word confessions" about the absence of sin in their lives, hoping these problems inside of them will go away. They walk around hoping nobody around them notices that they have these issues because it is not allowed. However, because of this way of thinking, they are now stuck. Because to acknowledge that they have sin within, that would be a negative confession. This is not a correct mindset to have about sin. Acknowledging that we have sin within us is not a negative confession—it is a statement of honesty.

SPIRITUAL DEFECTS

As a pastor, people come to me for ministry who have evil within them. I do not have a sign out here that says, "Be sure you have dealt with your sins first before you come into this ministry." Nor is there a sign that says I will coddle them in their sin. I will not make people feel good about sin. I will not tell them I love them, smile at them, give them a hug, and tell them they are the best thing since peanut butter to make them feel better about sin issues in their lives. I cannot associate with evil. If people come bringing demons with them, I am going to love them. At the same time, I will drive those suckers out—but I am going to love them. We have become caught in a place of dishonesty through religion. Galatians 6:1 said it for me, "Brethren, if a man be overtaken in a fault."

Brethren, if a man be overtaken in a fault, ye which are spiritual, restore such an one in the spirit of meekness; considering thyself, lest thou also be tempted. Galatians 6:1 KJV

It says the word *brethren* or *brothers*. That would be another word for believer. If a man be overtaken in a fault—what is a fault? It is a spiritual defect. How can we have a spiritual defect if we are born again? It happens all the time. It is the reason people have repented for sin and have become freed through our church and ministry. I have an analogy regarding dealing with sin in our lives. Have we ever been around someone who had a booger at the end of their nose and pretended not to notice it? Does that help the person? They may not feel embarrassed now, but it is still there. I want to help people with their "spiritual boogers." If they have a problem in their lives, like a booger hanging off the end of their nose, pretending it is not there does not do away with it. It is still hanging, and everyone sees it. It is a flickering, lingering reality of their lives. May I tell them it is there without making them feel ashamed and embarrassed?

Years ago, I was in a large church that had a "holier than thou" attitude. There were certain exalted individuals, and others were treated as second-class citizens. The sheep in the congregation were the peasants, and the leadership were exalted. They had an elitist mindset that dictated their spirituality by their financial success. Some had a lot of money, and some were not rich and treated as spiritually second-rate citizens. In that church, the true test of spirituality was their success. If someone were to be a part of leadership in this church, they had to be a success, and they were the ones who had the "holy hands."

Eventually, that church split right down the middle, and 50% of the leadership was in the sin of adultery. They were committing the sin of literal, physical adultery, and God dealt with that issue. Unfortunately, that congregation has never totally recovered. So, when Paul talks about doing something he did not want to do, he admits he had spiritual problems. I am so grateful for his transparency. When I get that boy in heaven, I am going to hug him. I am going to say, "Paul, man, I'm grateful for your transparency. You were an apostle from the foundation of the world. God ordained you to be an apostle to the Gentiles, and you had sin in your life, and I am grateful you admitted it. God still used you despite your battles. You cast out devils, healed the sick, and changed the destiny of the world—the Gentile world of which I am a part. I'm going to hang out with you, mister sinner boy."

PROVISION FOR WEAKNESS

Now, it is important to balance my message to avoid falling into another trap. There is the danger that just because we come into a place of fellowship with our defects and problems, we do not want to condone sin as a way of life. It does not mean that God wants us to condone the defect and keep it as a part of us. If people are not careful, they will believe that I am teaching that I condone sin or that I condone keeping spiritual defects. I am not! God hates sin, and He says that we are to have hatred for sin and evil.

> *Ye that love the LORD, hate evil: he preserveth the souls of his saints; he delivereth them out of the hand of the wicked. Psalm 97:10 KJV*

But I learned something about God — despite that hatred for evil and sin, He has made provision for us. If He has made provision for us in our weakness, then I must make provision for others in their weakness as they make provision for me in my weakness. I asked a question to a member of my staff the other day. I said, "I wonder what you would be like around me if I ever made a mistake. What if I sinned? What if I got caught in the midst of a situation and blew it? Would you still love me? Would you still honor me, or would you become an enemy of this ministry just because I am not perfect?" I think this is a challenging question for all of us. What will we do with each other when we bump into our problems and blemishes? What are we going to do?

Here is what we need to do: we need to be transparent with one another. The Bible says, "Confess your faults one to another."

> *Confess your faults one to another, and pray one for another, that ye may be healed. The effectual fervent prayer of a righteous man availeth much. James 5:16 KJV*

But we do not do that because we are afraid of each other. Can I trust someone with my life? Can they trust me with theirs? Not just in our successes, but what if we fail one another in a significant way? I do not mean we will become outright evil in our actions toward one another; we may just have a moment of failure or weakness. In those moments, can I trust someone with my life even when mistakes are made?

I was once the Pastor at another church and I knew there were some problems there. Devils were causing trouble through certain individuals. Sometimes a kingdom, otherwise known as an agenda, develops within the kingdom. One example of such an agenda would be Korah and those who rose up against Moses.

> *[1]Now Korah, the son of Izhar, the son of Kohath, the son of Levi, and Dathan and Abiram, the sons of Eliab, and On, the son of Peleth, sons of Reuben, took men: [2]And they rose up before Moses,*

*with certain of the children of Israel,
two hundred and fifty princes of the
assembly, famous in the congregation,
men of renown: ³And they gathered
themselves together against Moses and
against Aaron, and said unto them, Ye
take too much upon you, seeing all the
congregation are holy, every one of
them, and the LORD is among them:
wherefore then lift ye up yourselves
above the congregation of the LORD?
Numbers 16:1-3 KJV*

When Korah and his group separated
themselves against Moses, God made it clear whom
He had chosen by the judgment that came next.

*And the earth opened her mouth, and
swallowed them up, and their houses,
and all the men that appertained unto
Korah, and all their goods. Numbers
16:32 KJV*

One day, I had a cup at the door. As everyone
walked in, I said, "Would you sup this with me?
Would you sup this cup with me?" They withdrew
from me as if I had the plague. When the service
started, and someone came in late, I would stop the
music. I would say, "Oh, excuse me, you are coming
in late. Would you sup this cup with me?" Nobody
would touch that cup. The reason is they knew where
I was coming from. Nobody took that cup from my
hand in that entire congregation. Not one person took
that cup and supped with me because their hearts

were exposed, and they knew it. They were against me, and I had exposed their intentions publicly. I knew what I was dealing with, and I wanted them to know I knew it too. Did I love them? Yes, I loved them. Did they try to hurt me and destroy me? Yes. Do I still love them? Yes. I would receive them if they repented, but they no longer wish to fellowship with me.

WHAT ARE WE GOING TO DO WITH SIN?

Now, let us return to the crux of our conversation. James 5 says that we are to confess our faults one to another so that we may be healed.

> *Confess your faults one to another, and pray one for another, that ye may be healed. The effectual fervent prayer of a righteous man availeth much. James 5:16 KJV*

Returning to Galatians 6:1, we need to care for one another and help to recover others. The sentence begins with, "If a man (or a woman) be overtaken in a fault," and it transitions to an interesting statement: "ye which are spiritual." However, based upon where the Scripture goes next, I would like to insert an important perspective to interpreting it. I would submit that it refers to those who *consider* themselves spiritual. I love the way this reads in the majority text, the King James Version, because it goes on to state, "considering thyself."

Therefore, I piece together this Scripture to say it this way: "Those of you who consider yourselves spiritual (you spiritual ones), restore such a one in a spirit of meekness, and consider yourself also lest you be tempted in like manner and fall away."

> *Brethren, if a man be overtaken in a fault, ye which are spiritual, restore such an one in the spirit of meekness; considering thyself, lest thou also be tempted. Galatians 6:1 KJV*

Romans 2 says what we accuse another of, we ourselves are. Do we really consider that what we accuse another of, we ourselves are guilty of? It is because we are doing the same things.

> *Therefore thou art inexcusable, O man, whosoever thou art that judgest: for wherein thou judgest another, thou condemnest thyself; for thou that judgest doest the same things. Romans 2:1 KJV*

A great example was a series of events that happened between Jimmy Swaggart and Marvin Gorman. Swaggart accused Gorman of having an extramarital affair, and after Gorman revealed that Swaggart also had sexual sins in his life. I do not mean to use their names, but it is public knowledge so I can speak on the subject openly. From what I understand, both men repented. I am not against

Jimmy Swaggart because of problems in his life; I believe he loves God, and he loves people. He just had a spiritual defect. And Marvin also had a spiritual defect. What do we do with men who have defects? We burn them at the stake. Is this the way we should behave? What are we going to do with Paul? He is confessing in Romans 7 that he has sin in his life. Are we going to quit reading Romans because Paul had sin? We would have to eliminate about 80% of the New Testament writings because he is the author. And what about King David? We read his psalms and sing his songs—but he was a sinner. He was an adulterer; he had a man murdered. However, even after his sin was revealed, he was still known and called a man after God's own heart.

> *And when he had removed him, he raised up unto them David to be their king; to whom also he gave their testimony, and said, I have found David the son of Jesse, a man after mine own heart, which shall fulfil all my will. Acts 13:22 KJV*

Do we have a few sinners here, being the people of God after God's own heart? The issue is not sin. The issue is, what are we going to do with it? I look at spiritual defects this way: I do not judge people based on their defects. I want to know what they are going to do with the defect. What are we going to do with sins in our lives? Are we going to hide them? Are we going to pretend they do not exist? Are we going to create a church that pretends there is no evil in the Church? I came out of one of those churches. What are we going to do with it? Instead, let us look at what it says in 1 John: that whosoever is born of God cannot sin.

> *Whosoever is born of God doth not commit sin; for his seed remaineth in him: and he cannot sin, because he is born of God. 1 John 3:9 KJV*

What are we going to do with that one? If we have sin in our lives, does it mean we are not born again? Is that what it means? If we want to take a Scripture out of context, that is exactly what it means. It also says whosoever sinneth is of the devil.

> *He that committeth sin is of the devil; for the devil sinneth from the beginning. For this purpose the Son of God was manifested, that he might destroy the works of the devil. 1 John 3:8 KJV*

If that position is true, there are a lot of Christians who are of the devil. Instead, I want to position these Scriptures as a plumb line. A plumb line defines north and south to build a solid foundation for building structures. These Scriptures are not meant to accuse us; they are not addressing us personally. These Scriptures define that sin is not of God, and if we follow God, we must be willing to repent for sin as God convicts us of it. A person may say, "Well, I do not commit adultery, and I am not fornicating with anyone." Are they involved in strife and jealousy, envy and backbiting? Do they cast a jaundiced eye in judging others? Those are all sins. Let he who is without sin cast the first stone.

> *So when they continued asking him, he lifted up himself, and said unto them, He that is without sin among you, let him first cast a stone at her. John 8:7 KJV*

We are all growing up in God, are we not? Perhaps some of us are just two rungs above the other in our spiritual journeys. And if we are only two rungs above another person, we can slow down a minute and reach back and grab that person behind us by the hand to keep pulling them along.

THE LAW OF GOD

God, in the person of Jesus Christ, came from heaven to a sinful Church, and He mixed in with them. He walked with them, talked with them, touched them, fed them, taught them, and died for them. If it was good enough for my Boss, it is good enough for me to do the same things. Did He uphold high expectations for us? Yes. We are to be children of God; no higher expectations are possible for us.

> *¹⁵For ye have not received the spirit of bondage again to fear; but ye have received the Spirit of adoption, whereby we cry, Abba, Father. ¹⁶The Spirit itself beareth witness with our spirit, that we are the children of God: Romans 8:15-16 KJV*

Does He condone evil? No. Does He have a perfect hatred for evil? Yes. Does He love all of us? Yes. Now, onto Romans 7:15, it says, "For that which I do I allow not: for what I would, that do I not; but what I hate, that (is what) do I."

> *For that which I do I allow not: for*
> *what I would, that do I not; but what I*
> *hate, that do I. Romans 7:15 KJV*

I am going to paraphrase the next Scripture to bring this subject into focus. If then, I do those things which I wish I would not do, I consent unto the law that is it good.

> *If then I do that which I would not, I*
> *consent unto the law that it is good.*
> *Romans 7:16 KJV*

What does this mean? Let us look at the Scriptures. They are the law of God and tell us what is right and what is wrong. In Hebrews 5:13-14, it says the sign of maturity for a Christian is that they have exercised their senses to discern both good and evil.

> *13For every one that useth milk is*
> *unskilful in the word of righteousness:*
> *for he is a babe. 14But strong meat*
> *belongeth to them that are of full age,*
> *even those who by reason of use have*
> *their senses exercised to discern both*
> *good and evil. Hebrews 5:13-14 KJV*

Are we supposed to discern good and evil in the world? If not there, where are we to discern good and evil? That leaves two options to discern evil: in ourselves or our neighbors. We are not supposed to spend our time discerning good and evil in our neighbor—leave those neighbors alone. Where does righteousness begin? In the heart of our neighbors or in our hearts? Who needs to get spiritual first, our neighbors or us? Discernment begins in ourselves. Let the Kingdom of God begin in us, personally. We cannot blame our neighbor for our unrighteousness. It is not going to fly with God.

If we try to blame our neighbor for our sin, God will not allow us to get away with it. What will we do when we get to heaven and stand at the Judgment Seat of Christ? It will not go well for us if we look at the Lord and, as He evaluates our lives, we say, "Well, it was John's fault, my wife's fault, my mother's fault, or my grandfather's fault that I did not overcome sin in my life. They prevented me from following You." Even if we say, "The devil made me do it," that will not fly with God. It is not proper English, but I must say that we will not get away with blaming others for the issues in our lives: "It ain't goin' to fly."

Chapter 3: Sanctification Without Condemnation

THE BODY OF SIN

Now that we have established the Biblical foundation of personal responsibility, can we begin to teach sanctification without condemnation? The key is not just to teach sanctification but to teach it without condemnation. I am a teacher of righteousness, but I am not a legalist. I do not come and hit someone over the head with truth or threaten them with death or hell to provoke them to repent.

The worst thing that could happen in this church and ministry is if I threaten someone and put them under condemnation for sin. Then they will pretend they are righteous, especially around me, so I do not see their problems and sins. I do not want people to act that way. If someone has devils, they need to be honest about them and not hide the problem. The Church is the best place for sin to manifest so we may address it. We can deal with it together. We love people. Just let it all hang out. We can deal with it. By spiritual discernment, a gift of the Holy Spirit, we are able to separate people from evil. As Scripture says, "It is no more I that do it, but sin that dwelleth in me."

> *Now then it is no more I that do it, but sin that dwelleth in me. Romans 7:17 KJV*

When Paul says it is no longer him that does it — this is an important distinction that I must point out. When we fall into sin, we buy a lie from Satan's kingdom. And as we commit to performing sin, we are no longer the ones sinning, but a being known as "sin" manifests through us. These are evil spirits who manifest through us as humans. The problem is that many people in the Church have been taught these Scriptures are metaphors and symbols. They do not believe a literal being known as *sin* is manifesting through Paul. At the same time, when they look at other Scriptures, such as 2 Timothy 1:7, they do not consider what it is truly saying.

> *For God hath not given us the spirit of fear; but of power, and of love, and of a sound mind. 2 Timothy 1:7 KJV*

When it says that God has not given us the spirit of fear, this is not metaphorical language. It is a literal evil spirit of fear. What Spirit has Father God given us? The Holy Spirit. He gives us the power, love, and soundness of mind that only the Godhead can impart to us. So when evil spirits known as the body of sin tempt us, and we fall into sin, they manifest through us, and we are led into captivity to them.

> *Knowing this, that our old man is crucified with him, that the body of sin*

might be destroyed, that henceforth we
should not serve sin. Romans 6:6 KJV

SEPARATION

An essential role of ministry is to lead a person
to repentance around a spirit of fear. After
repentance, the minister casts out the evil spirit of
fear. Then the process of sanctification begins as the
person is released to think, speak, and act according
to faith in an area where they were once bound.

God is able to separate us from areas where we
are bound. He cares for us despite the sin in our lives.
He saw our sin, but He saved us, and He loves us. He
released the Holy Spirit to live in us despite sin in our
lives. Do we think the Holy Spirit can live in the same
place evil can live? I hear this line of reasoning, "Well,
the Holy Spirit and the devil cannot exist at the same
place at the same time." Where did they get that idea?
Is there a Scripture that proves their point? There is
no proof. So where did they come up with it? They
just had a thought one day. We have to watch out for
our thoughts. If they do not match the Word of God,
they are not valid. As I like to say, they are kind of
"squirrelly" and "full of nuts".

Now, is the Holy Spirit in the earth today? Yes.
Who else is in the earth today? The devil. In Job 1,
when the sons of God came to present themselves
before the Lord, Satan came with them.

*Now there was a day when the sons of
God came to present themselves before
the LORD, and Satan came also among
them. Job 1:6 KJV*

Was he, Satan, there before the Lord? Were
they there at the same place? Yes. There is a battle on
this planet for our lives and our sanity. The choice is
ours to make. Will we choose to follow Father God, or
will we choose to follow Satan's kingdom? Each
kingdom will form us depending on which one we
follow. One Kingdom will form us according to
righteousness and the other kingdom according to
unrighteousness.

Moving on, let us go to Zechariah 3:1.

*And he shewed me Joshua the high
priest standing before the angel of the
LORD, and Satan standing at his right
hand to resist him. Zechariah 3:1 KJV*

I will break down this Scripture part by part to
help us understand what it says. It says, "And he
shewed me Joshua the high priest standing before the
angel of the LORD, and Satan standing at his right
hand to resist him." Who is standing there? Joshua.
And who is there who is invisible to Joshua? The
angel of the Lord and Satan. Now these beings,
invisible to Joshua, are all at the same place with him.

However, Joshua, the high priest, was not in
heaven. He was standing on the earth as the high
priest over Israel. And who was invisible with him

right there on earth? The angel of the Lord. Who else was there? Satan was there, but he was disembodied. Why would I use the term "disembodied" to describe Satan? Disembodied means he does not have a physical body. That is why he will need the human male, known as the anti-Christ, to carry out his plans in the future. That is also why he needed a serpent to speak to Adam and Eve, and that is why he needs us to manifest his evil nature on this planet today. He has no access to this physical world except through a physical human being or some other physical creature. For emphasis, I want to repeat that Satan and evil spirits have no access to this physical world that God created for us unless he uses one of us as a medium. He is invisible around the edges of creation, looking for a way in to influence humanity through thoughts. So who is there with the angel of the Lord and Joshua? Satan.

And then the Lord spoke to Satan.

> *²And the LORD said unto Satan, The LORD rebuke thee, O Satan; even the LORD that hath chosen Jerusalem rebuke thee: is not this a brand plucked out of the fire? ³Now Joshua was clothed with filthy garments, and stood before the angel. ⁴And he answered and spake unto those that stood before him, saying, Take away the filthy garments from him. And unto him he said, Behold, I have caused thine iniquity to pass from thee, and I will clothe thee with change of raiment. ⁵And I said, Let them*

set a fair mitre upon his head. So they
set a fair mitre upon his head, and
clothed him with garments. And the
angel of the LORD stood by. Zechariah
3:2-5 KJV

They were talking about Joshua, the high priest. They were speaking over him at the same place at the same time. I am bringing this to our attention because when the Holy Spirit came to awaken our spirits unto God, evil spirits in our lives did not disappear. The Holy Spirit dwells within us, and He lives in the midst of the devils in our lives. Some suggest we have a new, different spirit when we are born again. That is not the case. The day we were born again, we still had the same spirit, the same soul, and the same body as we did before that point in our lives. The first aspect of our lives that changed was that our spirits came alive to God as a work of the Holy Spirit. We were living life alone and now we are no longer alone. Greater is He who is in us than he who is in the world.

Ye are of God, little children, and have
overcome them: because greater is he
that is in you, than he that is in the
world. 1 John 4:4 KJV

And now we have the Holy Spirit who has come into our lives and will lead us into all truth.

Howbeit when he, the Spirit of truth, is
come, he will guide you into all truth:
for he shall not speak of himself; but

whatsoever he shall hear, that shall he
speak: and he will shew you things to
come. John 16:13 KJV

THE RENEWAL OF OUR MINDS

When we were born again, how did our minds change? To understand our minds, it is crucial to define them accurately. Another Biblical term for our mind is our soul, which would include our memory. Who we are as human beings, even the evil parts of us from the past, remain with us forever. We never lose our memory; that is a recollection of our lives. That is a record of who we are. The events we remember have been part of our existence, retained in our souls. As a physical human being, who we are is found within the realm of our minds or our souls. So, how are our souls renewed? "With the washing of water by the word."

> *²⁶That he might sanctify and cleanse it*
> *with the washing of water by the word,*
> *²⁷That he might present it to himself a*
> *glorious church, not having spot, or*
> *wrinkle, or any such thing; but that it*
> *should be holy and without blemish.*
> *Ephesians 5:26-27 KJV*

What does the Word of God do? The Word brings a thought into our thinking that is different from the thinking we had in the past. Before, our mindset was formed after the thinking of Satan and his ways of thinking. Now, as we read the Bible, our mind is open to a new life and a new way of thinking. We have the Word of God to compare to the old way of thinking in order to reevaluate it. We can repent of this "stinking thinking," and we have new ideas coming from Scripture to inform our future decisions. We are now able to inspect both types of thinking in our mind at the same time.

LONG-TERM MEMORY

There is a specific part of the soul we need to address: the subject of long-term memory. If we meet up with someone today, our minds will take a mental picture of them. For some of us, it will be stored as a short-term memory. For others of us, it will become a long-term memory. If someone were to meet me, I might just be a passing vapor in their life, and they will forget me. Others might lock into me at some dimension. Something that I say or do becomes memorable because it impacts them. If I leave an impact, they will remember something about me forever. It might not always be a good memory, but they will remember something about me forever.

Our minds are taking pictures all the time. Our eyes are cameras that take pictures; we are listening with our ears and experiencing the world with our five physical senses. Our brains are instantly taking pictures by the millions, which are electrochemical. It is an electrochemical occurrence that uses an electrical chemical in our brain cells to mirror the image of what we just heard, saw, tasted, smelled, or touched. In our long-term memory, our brains go through another stage called protein synthesis. My understanding is that, in protein synthesis, there is a component of our genetics that plays a role in the process known as RNA. This component of RNA takes the electrochemical picture and integrates it into our brain cells permanently as a part of our memory. The image, biologically, becomes a part of us, not just a mirror image stored somewhere.

When we minister to people who need healing from past traumas, we have to keep in mind the role of long-term memory in their journeys. Even if I deal with the human spirit in teaching a person and cast out the evil spirits that have taken advantage of their past trauma, they can still have the same thoughts of an evil spirit without an evil spirit present. Through traumas and patterns of the past, an evil spirit has programmed them to think like an evil spirit. Even when an evil spirit is cast out, the mind can have the very same memories it gave us in the past.

This is where I believe people who promote inner healing miss the target. Inner healing focuses on the healing of memories, but that does not remove the core problem. I am focused on the removal of the evil spirit that joins a person in a traumatic event and then the renewal of the mind. So I do not practice inner healing. I am not a disciple of various practitioners of it. I know some of them personally and have known them for years. However, I am not interested in changing people's memories. I have observed people who came to grip with their past memories, but they were still tormented in their inner man. I want to

ensure that we are cleansed on both dimensions—
soul and spirit, not just one. Even if the evil spirit
representing that victimization and tragedy is
removed, the mind must be renewed according to the
Word of God.

> *²⁶That he might sanctify and cleanse it*
> *with the washing of water by the word,*
> *²⁷That he might present it to himself a*
> *glorious church, not having spot, or*
> *wrinkle, or any such thing; but that it*
> *should be holy and without blemish.*
> *Ephesians 5:26-27 KJV*

The good fruit coming from this ministry is
freedom from torment that people are experiencing.
When they repent, and the evil spirit is cast out, we
find these individuals are being healed. At the same
time, their memories have not been altered, and they
still remember the tragedies of the past. We always
will, but we do not have the pain that accompanied
those memories. As for those who teach those
memories of the past may be removed, they are
manipulating the soul and getting people to live in
denial. And I will be bluntly honest, in ministry, my
purpose is to help people to come out of denial
because when they suppress a traumatic memory or
issue, they open the door for an evil spirit. All
suppression of memories opens the door for an evil
spirit to help to suppress them. However, behind the
denial and suppression, an evil spirit torments them
forever until they face the issue bringing the torment
into their lives. I have recognized it in the past, and I

recognize it working in people today; I am not deceived.

UNDER CONSTRUCTION

My point is to bring all memories into focus. Now, I know there are Scriptures that teach us to leave those things that are behind and stop dwelling on the past.

> *[13]Brethren, I count not myself to have apprehended: but this one thing I do, forgetting those things which are behind, and reaching forth unto those things which are before, [14]I press toward the mark for the prize of the high calling of God in Christ Jesus. Philippians 3:13-14 KJV*

Scripture also states that we are a new creature and all things are new.

> *Therefore if any man be in Christ, he is a new creature: old things are passed away; behold, all things are become new. 2 Corinthians 5:17 KJV*

But wait a minute. Just because we are pressing on into the future does not mean our enemy does not exist. When we became born again, were we immune to temptation? When we became born again, were we immune to the devil? When we became born again, were we immune to sin? Are we not still capable of sinning? However, we can become stuck because of what I have termed "black-and-white thinking." We are all a shade of gray because we have sin in our lives. If God is light and all goodness and Satan represents darkness—we are somewhere in-between. Some of us are a lighter shade of gray, and others of us are a darker shade. If we perceive Scripture through this lens, we will hyperventilate, freak out, and become fearful when reading certain passages. For instance, the Bible says whosoever is born of God cannot sin.

> *Whosoever is born of God doth not*
> *commit sin; for his seed remaineth in*
> *him: and he cannot sin, because he is*
> *born of God. 1 John 3:9 KJV*

"Black-and-white thinking" will cause a person to interpret this Scripture in extreme ways. It will tempt them to live in denial because every human has sin in their lives. They want to be a child of God but believe they cannot be if they live in an "all-or-nothing" mindset. They are not considering that we are all on a journey of faith. As I like to say, I am under construction. I am not who I was in the past, and I am not who I will be in the future. I am growing up day by day as I repent for sin and learn to follow God according to His Word.

PRESENT PROGRESSIVE

As I studied Scripture, I came to understand a concept concerning our journey of identity. It is a grammar term known as *present progressive,* as discussed in chapter one. If we go back to 2 Corinthians 5:17, we will find an example of present progressive in Scripture.

> *Therefore if any man be in Christ, he is a new creature: old things are passed away; behold, all things are become new. 2 Corinthians 5:17 KJV*

At the end of the verse, it says, "behold, all things are become new." If we are paying attention, this phrase may seem awkward and improper use of the English language. However, it does not say that all things have become new as a past tense event. It says that all things are becoming new — this is an example of present progressive. We are progressing in the present toward an end. We are growing and being formed.

Most of our journey as believers is present progressive. What is faith? Present progressive. Are we working out our salvation daily? That is present progressive. Are we all that we believe we should be in the new birth, or are we being reformed by God? It is a present progressive process. Are all the promises of God ours in the present, or are we trusting God that they will come to pass in the future? Are we walking in all of them yet? Why not? Because we are living in a present progressive state. Have we achieved all the blessings of God in our lives? Have we seen all the healing, deliverance, and fulfillment of promises yet? No. But what are we doing? We are in the present progressive process of appropriating them to our lives.

The degree of our sanctification is the degree of our blessings. Our blessings are in direct relationship to our obedience. If we are unwilling to acknowledge and repent for sin in our lives, we are living in disobedience to Scripture, which will not lead to blessing. However, some in the Church teach a route to blessings without obedience, and it is not working. In the Word of Faith movement, the charismatic movement, the Pentecostal movement, and many other movements, there are believers still demonized and sick despite the promise of blessings. God help us. Now, that is not an indictment. To those who are part of those movements reading this, I must add there are many other denominations in worse shape that do not even teach promise. The positive aspect of the Word of Faith and charismatic movements is that they are still trying to teach that God heals and delivers today — and God bless them in that endeavor. However, many of them do not understand the connection between disease and sin. In fact, there are those who will teach that there is no connection between the spirit of man and the physical dimension of man as if our spirituality has no impact on our sanity, peace, and physical health.

THE CONNECTION BETWEEN OUR SPIRIT AND BODY

Some people teach that there is no connection between the spirit of man and the physical connection, yet Proverbs 17:22 says, "a broken spirit drieth the bones."

A merry heart doeth good like a medicine: but a broken spirit drieth the bones. Proverbs 17:22 KJV

It also says in Scripture that the spirit of man shall sustain him in his infirmity.

The spirit of a man will sustain his infirmity; but a wounded spirit who can bear? Proverbs 18:14 KJV

In these two Scriptures, we have a connection between the spirit of man and our physical condition — the health or disease of our bodies.

BIND THE STRONG MAN

However, before moving on to another subject, I want to address suppressed memories related to trauma. Someone might have a question in the area of healing and deliverance: do the suppressed memories have to be exposed and dealt with? Generally, yes, they do. At the same time, it does not mean that every single memory must be dealt with, but there is a class of healing that requires addressing certain types of demonics. We approach ministry not from specific demons but from a class of bondage. We address levels of bondage and categories of bondage. Sometimes when a class of bondage is defeated, everything under it is removed, and a person is healed because the power of it is broken. For example, in the area of an Unloving spirit, if I can bring a person to a place where they are able to receive love without fear, there are legions of demons that are broken in their life forever.

By breaking their power, I mean to say that a person is no longer deceived by lies from Satan's kingdom in this area of their lives. As a result of this change to a person's spirituality and mindset, the evil spirits are no longer able to torment and control them. Because of the work of the Holy Spirit to deliver and teach a person, the evil spirits' power is broken off of them. In those cases, a positive floodgate opens up, and these evil spirits are gone without having to get involved with specific underlying spirits. There is a five-layered kingdom that we are dealing with in ministry. There is a hierarchy of bureaucracy of Satan's kingdom, and if we are not careful, we will be chasing the fruit of the problem rather than the root spiritual issues. I do not go down a demon list. I have seen ministries go down demon lists, and we are not going there.

We look at bondage from the standpoint of classes of bondage. The Bible says we should bind or take spiritual authority over the strong man so that we can spoil his house. What is "his house?" It is any area of a person's life that that spirit is operating unhindered in its evil nature.

> *28 But if I cast out devils by the Spirit of God, then the kingdom of God is come unto you. 29Or else how can one enter into a strong man's house, and spoil his goods, except he first bind the strong man? and then he will spoil his house. Matthew 12:28-29 KJV*

In ministry, we are looking at classes. We are discerning classes of bondage and disease, both psychological and biological, which represent a phylum and a subphylum of demonic powers. In school, they teach certain principles of zoology. Part of zoology is the categorization of creation, such as phylum and subphylum. The phylum and subphylum of zoology include all those long words and terms that are hard to pronounce. In Satan's kingdom, there are phylum and subphylum. Ephesians 6 lays out the organization of Satan's kingdom. It says our battle is not against flesh and blood but against principalities and powers, the rulers of the darkness of this world, and spiritual wickedness in high places.

> *For we wrestle not against flesh and blood, but against principalities, against powers, against the rulers of the darkness of this world, against spiritual wickedness in high places. Ephesians 6:12 KJV*

And there, we have a four-tiered structure. The head of the four-tiered structure is Satan himself. We refer to the location of Satan's kingdom as the second heaven. This is not a label found in the Bible, but is it an inference I have made based upon known information from Scriptures. The Bible specifically refers to the current world we live in as the first heaven and the first earth. It is where physical creation exists.

And I saw a new heaven and a new earth: for the first heaven and the first earth were passed away; and there was no more sea. Revelation 21:1 KJV

Contrary to certain ideas in Christianity, I find no evidence of a seventh heaven. However, the Scripture does describe the third heaven as the dimension where God lives. It is not a physical dimension we see with our physical eyes.

[2]I knew a man in Christ above fourteen years ago, (whether in the body, I cannot tell; or whether out of the body, I cannot tell: God knoweth;) such an one caught up to the third heaven. [3]And I knew such a man, (whether in the body, or out of the body, I cannot tell: God knoweth;) [4]How that he was caught up into paradise, and heard unspeakable words, which it is not lawful for a man to utter. 2 Corinthians 12:2-4 KJV

While Scriptures do not refer to a second heaven, because I have found a first and third, I have inferred the other spiritual dimension described in Scripture would be the "second heaven" or a separate dimension we cannot see with our eyes that is separate from the third heaven. In Scripture, the spiritual dimension is called the "dry place." When an evil spirit is cast out, it is cast into a dry place. It is not a physical location but a spiritual location separate from God.

When the unclean spirit is gone out of a man, he walketh through dry places, seeking rest; and finding none, he saith, I will return unto my house whence I came out. Luke 11:24 KJV

As mentioned previously, if anyone is interested in the in-depth explanation, it can be found in my teaching on Spirit World Realities. In this teaching on Spirit World Realities, we address what sin is, where it comes from, where it is today, and what it is doing. I have taken a firm position in ministry that sin is not a concept. It is not even a state of being; it is a being. There are sinful beings and obedient beings.

Chapter 4: Sin is Not Our Identity

WHEN WE DO WHAT WE HATE

The importance of addressing sin is to bring us back to the subject of our spirituality and its connection to our physical well-being. Romans 7:16 says, "If then I do that which I would not, I consent unto the law that it is good."

> *If then I do that which I would not, I consent unto the law that it is good.*
> *Romans 7:16 KJV*

Let us break apart this Scripture. The law listed in this Scripture is the law of God. This is not a reference just to the Law of Moses found in the Torah, but the law in this Scripture refers to the entire Word of God. What the Bible has said about our existence, good and evil, is the road map for sanity. Paul is saying here that he has a problem. In fact, going back to verse 15, Paul says that the things he hates, that is what he does.

> *For that which I do I allow not: for what I would, that do I not; but what I hate, that do I. Romans 7:15 KJV*

He basically says in verse 16, "If I do those things that I hate, I consent by my words and actions unto the Word of God that the evil law I am now following is actually good and truth. Additionally, by my actions and words of disobedience, I am saying God's Word is evil and not truth." Another example is when the Bible says if we, from our hearts, do not forgive our brother his trespass, our Father in heaven shall not forgive us ours.

> *[14]For if ye forgive men their trespasses, your heavenly Father will also forgive you: [15]But if ye forgive not men their trespasses, neither will your Father forgive your trespasses. Matthew 6:14-15 KJV*

If I go into unforgiveness, and I am not going to forgive people for what they did to me, then I am consenting unto this new law of unforgiveness that the law of God concerning forgiveness is evil and this new law is good. That makes Satan's words truth unto me, except that I am now following a lie. And that lie is the new "word" I am following. This makes it the new concept or mindset I am now following.

So Paul is saying here that when he does those things that he hates, he is affirming certain principles by his actions. The new law, contrary to the Word of God, that is causing him to do these things that he hated is forming a new law in his life. So this new law becomes a "thus saith the Lord" unto us when we rebel against Father God.

WHICH LAW ARE WE ESTABLISHING?

Rather than following Father God, we are establishing the opposite. Instead of loving our brother, we hate our brother. Well, perhaps not all of them; just specific individuals. When we pick and choose whom to love and whom to hate, we have a leavened word. Someone might say, "I forgive everyone." However, the person listening may respond, "What about John?" Their response may sound like, "Well, I am working on it." What does that phrase "working on it" mean? Perhaps, we reason that we will choose to forgive one day. However, in practice, we are following another law through our decision not to forgive John for what he has done to us.

The Word of God does not allow us the option to forgive our brother when we feel like it and remain in unforgiveness because we are "working on it." To leaven the Word of God is to change Scripture by adding to or removing from what it says. Deciding what we will follow and what we will disregard from the Bible makes the Word of God evil unto us, and the rebellion we are following good unto us.

Woe unto them that call evil good, and good evil; that put darkness for light, and light for darkness; that put bitter for sweet, and sweet for bitter! Isaiah 5:20 KJV

That is how Satan rules us. This is also why he is called the "god of this world".

*In whom the god of this world hath
blinded the minds of them which believe
not, lest the light of the glorious gospel
of Christ, who is the image of God,
should shine unto them. 2 Corinthians
4:4 KJV*

He controls men through their minds. How
does God work with us? By renewing our minds
through the washing of the water of the Word.

*²⁵Husbands, love your wives, even as
Christ also loved the church, and gave
himself for it; ²⁶That he might sanctify
and cleanse it with the washing of
water by the word, Ephesians 5:25-26
KJV*

Jesus tells us that if we love Him, we will keep
his commandments.

*If ye love me, keep my commandments.
John 14:15 KJV*

But what do some people perceive when they
read that Scripture? They may see, "If you love me,
you will be a slave unto my commandments." With
that perception, they push away God saying,
"Nobody is going to tell me what to do; bless God." If
someone thinks that way, they have an anti-Christ
spirit. They are in rebellion, and rebellion is as the sin
of witchcraft, according to 1 Samuel 15:23.

²⁵Husbands, love your wives, even as Christ also loved the church, and gave himself for it; ²⁶That he might sanctify and cleanse it with the washing of water by the word, ²⁷That he might present it to himself a glorious church, not having spot, or wrinkle, or any such thing; but that it should be holy and without blemish. ²⁸So ought men to love their wives as their own bodies. He that loveth his wife loveth himself. ²⁹For no man ever yet hated his own flesh; but nourisheth and cherisheth it, even as the Lord the church: ³⁰For we are members of his body, of his flesh, and of his bones. Ephesians 5:25-30 KJV

Jesus is my husband, and I am learning to be a good wife. I am learning how to be a better one. As I learn how to be a better wife to Christ, I can be a better husband to my wife. I cannot be a good husband to my wife if I am not learning to be a good wife to Christ. So I am learning how to be a good wife, and my wife is reaping the benefits of that. I am also learning how to love my Father in heaven, and that is making me a better father to my children. I have some generational iniquity to work out.

Some contend that once we are born again, we are not just forgiven of our sins, but we do not carry the baggage of the past, including the sins of past generations. Unfortunately, in ministry, we have found too many examples of people who think and behave like their carnal generations after becoming a born-again believers. Their patterns of thought and behavior do not reflect the "mind of Christ".

GENERATIONAL INIQUITY

In Scriptures, I have a found examples of generational iniquity plainly described in Exodus.

> *⁵Thou shalt not bow down thyself to them, nor serve them: for I the LORD thy God am a jealous God, visiting the iniquity of the fathers upon the children unto the third and fourth generation of them that hate me; ⁶And shewing mercy unto thousands of them that love me, and keep my commandments. Exodus 20:5-6 KJV*

Someone may think they do not hate God, but as I established earlier, if we disobey the Word of God, we are not loving God. In other words, if we disobey God, we are, in essence, hating God. This is not entire, but we are opposed to God and His ways in that area. Doing that will lead to a generational iniquity that will be passed from generation to generation. Indeed, when we were born again, we were forgiven of our sins, but might I ask: did we stop sinning after that event? If we are honest, the answer is "no". There are areas of our lives where we still struggle with sin after being born again because we have been trained by sin in our families. It is part of our soul and mind as much as it is a part of our spirituality.

May I show an example from Scripture of a family who struggled with lying? They loved God, but in this specific area, multiple generations fell into this sin. As Exodus states, we see the iniquity visited to the third and fourth generation.

> *Thou shalt not bow down thyself to them, nor serve them: for I the LORD thy God am a jealous God, visiting the iniquity of the fathers upon the children unto the third and fourth generation of them that hate me; Exodus 20:4 KJV*

Abraham had a lying spirit and fear of man as exemplified by Scripture. When he was confronted by Pharaoh concerning his wife, he lied that she was not his wife but his sister to avoid being killed.

> *[11]And it came to pass, when he was come near to enter into Egypt, that he said unto Sarai his wife, Behold now, I know that thou art a fair woman to look upon: [12]Therefore it shall come to pass, when the Egyptians shall see thee, that they shall say, This is his wife: and they will kill me, but they will save thee alive. [13]Say, I pray thee, thou art my sister: that it may be well with me for thy sake; and my soul shall live because of thee. Genesis 12:11-13 KJV*

His son Isaac said almost the exact words and logic as his father, Abraham. Did this logic come from

God or Satan? It was Satan's kingdom that inspired him to lie.

> *⁶And Isaac dwelt in Gerar: ⁷And the men of the place asked him of his wife; and he said, She is my sister: for he feared to say, She is my wife; lest, said he, the men of the place should kill me for Rebekah; because she was fair to look upon. Genesis 26:6-7 KJV*

This pattern of lying extended into the next two generations as Isaac's son, Jacob, deceived his father to receive the blessing. Jacob's sons also lied to him concerning the death of their brother, Joseph. That would be four generations of liars. Does that entirely remove any righteousness from their lives? No. However, if left unrepented, these sins will extend from generation to generation. Therefore, the Word of God is used to examine our lives, including in the area of our families and our spouse's families.

My ancestors did not take care of their wives and children. My ancestors destroyed and brutally oppressed their wives and children. I have had some generational sin issues to work out in my life that I inherited. We all do.

THE SIN WITHIN

Going back to Romans 7:16, it says Paul does those things that he wished he would not do, and this was consenting unto the Word of God that this new law (that is making him do the things he wished he would not do) is actually good.

> *If then I do that which I would not, I consent unto the law that it is good. Romans 7:16 KJV*

Now, let us go to verse 17. Paul says, "Now then it is no more I that do it." What is he doing? The evil. And it says, "The sin that dwelleth in me." The sin that dwelled in him did not dwell on the tree next door to his house, shooting fiery darts at him at 100 miles an hour. How can that be in this born-again, filled-with-the-Holy-Ghost apostle?

> *Now then it is no more I that do it, but sin that dwelleth in me. Romans 7:17 KJV*

Remember, the question is not what died; rather, it is what came alive? As we continue to read, we will find out Paul came alive. However, it is important to note that when we study the Pauline Epistles, he teaches us the circumcision of the flesh. This circumcision is the cutting away of the sin that dwells within, and that is the crux of sanctification.

> *For we are the circumcision, which worship God in the spirit, and rejoice in Christ Jesus, and have no confidence in the flesh. Philippians 3:3 KJV*

A NEW CREATURE?

In Christianity, some teach we are a new creature and a new creation and that it is an entirely completed process. What they have done is taken the promise of faith, and they have determined it has already come to pass prematurely. What they have done is seen that by the promise of faith, we are a new creation and a new creature, but they do not make a place for the process of growth in the meantime. We are still groaning with the rest of the world in our torment. The Word says the whole creation groans, and we also groan with it in pain.

> ¹⁹*For the earnest expectation of the creature waiteth for the manifestation of the sons of God.* ²⁰*For the creature was made subject to vanity, not willingly, but by reason of him who hath subjected the same in hope,* ²¹*Because the creature itself also shall be delivered from the bondage of corruption into the glorious liberty of the children of God.* ²²*For we know that the whole creation groaneth and travaileth in pain together until now.* Romans 8:19-22 KJV*

Has the "earnest expectation" of faith been fulfilled already? No. So, when we are a new creature, we have come alive to God. We are not as we shall be, but in the twinkling of an eye, we shall be changed.

> *In a moment, in the twinkling of an eye, at the last trump: for the trumpet shall*

*sound, and the dead shall be raised
incorruptible, and we shall be changed.
1 Corinthians 15:52 KJV*

When will this happen? In the First
Resurrection. What is the First Resurrection? It is the
resurrection of those who have died before the 1000-
year reign of Christ. This would be the resurrection of
believers because they are those who will reign with
Christ. Therefore, being part of the First Resurrection
will be a blessing.

> *⁴And I saw thrones, and they sat upon
> them, and judgment was given unto
> them: and I saw the souls of them that
> were beheaded for the witness of Jesus,
> and for the word of God, and which had
> not worshipped the beast, neither his
> image, neither had received his mark
> upon their foreheads, or in their hands;
> and they lived and reigned with Christ a
> thousand years. ⁵But the rest of the dead
> lived not again until the thousand years
> were finished. This is the first
> resurrection. ⁶Blessed and holy is he
> that hath part in the first resurrection:
> on such the second death hath no power,
> but they shall be priests of God and of
> Christ, and shall reign with him a
> thousand years. Revelation 20:4-6 KJV*

The Church is becoming confused and insane
over teachings that indicate the promises, and even
the First Resurrection, have already happened. We

have not yet been changed. In the future, we will be changed in the twinkling of an eye. By faith, we are now alive to God when before we were dead to God. We are establishing the Kingdom of God by our obedience despite the devil; this is a miracle. Our obedience to Father God is an absolute kick in the teeth of Satan, the god of this world.

> *In whom the god of this world hath blinded the minds of them which believe not, lest the light of the glorious gospel of Christ, who is the image of God, should shine unto them. 2 Corinthians 4:4 KJV*

I, Henry, choose not to sin when there is every reason to, with temptation all around me. And when I do so, I repent when I sin against God. Satan, who was perfect in his ways from the day he was created, fell. When he was known as Lucifer or Helel, from the Hebrew in the Strong's Concordance, he rebelled against Father God.

> *How art thou fallen from heaven, O Lucifer, son of the morning! how art thou cut down to the ground, which didst weaken the nations! Isaiah 14:12 KJV*

However, he was not created evil. He was perfect in his ways the day he was created until he sinned and did not repent. He did not repent to Father God for his rebellion.

¹⁴Thou art the anointed cherub that covereth; and I have set thee so: thou wast upon the holy mountain of God; thou hast walked up and down in the midst of the stones of fire. ¹⁵Thou wast perfect in thy ways from the day that thou wast created, till iniquity was found in thee. Ezekiel 28:14-15 KJV

Now, we are a new creature in Christ Jesus. The old things have passed away; behold, all things are becoming new.

Therefore if any man be in Christ, he is a new creature: old things are passed away; behold, all things are become new. 2 Corinthians 5:17 KJV

My eyes are wide open. I know what Henry Wright should not be, and I know what Henry Wright should be in the mind of God. This is where the Holy Spirit has come to sanctify me, purge me of sin, and make me a vessel of honor. He is still working me over really well. I have about 14 or 15 different major areas of my life under reconstruction all the time. Because many people have taken the promise of faith and have brought it to an immediate conclusion, the Church is confused. They teach us to believe more in order to become more of what the Bible promises. The problem is they have not considered sanctification. If our journey is already completed, then we do not have any need for sanctification. We already are what we need to be; we just need to walk in it.

Well, in a way, that is correct. But we are trying to walk in something while bringing the baggage of sin with us. No, God wants us to stop, make a little pile here, and make a little pile there. Dropping the weight of sin so we can walk more freely every day. The Church is burdened with itself because discernment has not been taught. All that we have been taught is promise. The promises of God are yea and nay, but promise without discernment is still bondage, and the Church is in bondage. The Church is sick.

I read an article the other day that was left on my desk by a pastor of some denomination that said we are to accept disease because healing will be in the First Resurrection. He said, "Do not worry about it, you will be getting a new body any day, even if you are stuck with the diseases you have today." If that was the case, why did Jesus come and heal anybody? If this position were true, Jesus would have just said, "Hey, believe on Me and in the First Resurrection, you will be free of disease." He did not do that. He healed them of their diseases and cast out their evil spirits.

In verse 17 of Romans 7, it says, "Now then it is no more I that do it, but sin that dwelleth in me."

Now then it is no more I that do it, but sin that dwelleth in me. Romans 7:17 KJV

In verse 17, where does sin dwell? In him. Paul, who was born again, had sin dwelling in him. What are we going to do with that, Church? What are we going to do with that fact? Overlook it? That is exactly what a lot of the Church does. Well, that was Paul's observation. In verse 18, he goes on to say, "For I know that in me (that is, in my flesh) dwelleth no good thing: for to will is present with me." This flesh is not talking about his human body, by the way.

> *For I know that in me (that is, in my flesh,) dwelleth no good thing: for to will is present with me; but how to perform that which is good I find not. Romans 7:18 KJV*

The word *flesh* has two components: the first part is the indwelling presence of evil spirits by their nature, and the second is our unrenewed minds that have been programmed with thoughts from evil spirits through past experiences. Both dimensions need to be cleansed. Remember what I quoted from 2 Corinthians 7:1? It says, "Having therefore these promises, dearly beloved, let us cleanse ourselves from all filthiness of the flesh and spirit."

> *Having therefore these promises, dearly beloved, let us cleanse ourselves from all filthiness of the flesh and spirit, perfecting holiness in the fear of God. 2 Corinthians 7:1 KJV*

That does not mean we need to take a shower. Cleanse ourselves of all filthiness of the flesh does not mean our bodies are physically dirty. Do we think Paul is telling someone to take a shower? No. Do we believe the "circumcision of the heart" refers to physical heart surgery? No. What is the circumcision of the heart? What are we cutting away? The heart is the heart of man which is the spirit of man, not the soul. So what are we cutting away? Evil spirits from our human spirit. The human spirit is the location of evil spirits that torment us. If we have a spirit of fear, it resides in our human spirit because it is a spirit. Evil spirits are spirit and they reside in our human spirit. Naturally, if we are comparing like with like, spirit is with spirit, and human body with human body. God, the Holy Spirit, is a Spirit. Where does He live—in our mind or our body? Neither of them. The Holy Spirit lives in our human spirit.

UNRIGHTEOUSNESS MANIFESTS

If Satan and his kingdom are disembodied spirits, how can they access us? They have access to us through the spirit dimension. They also have access to us through our five physical senses to program us in our thinking so they may have access to our human spirit. I am not teaching extensively on the topic of demonology. That is not our purpose here. Romans 7:18 says, "For I know that in me (that is, in my flesh,) dwelleth no good thing: for to will is present with me; but how to perform that which is good I find not."

For I know that in me (that is, in my flesh,) dwelleth no good thing: for to

will is present with me; but how to
perform that which is good I find not.
Romans 7:18 KJV

As a Christian, have we ever been known to do good works? More than likely, we have been taught righteousness from many teachers and pastors. However, are we able to walk in it all the time? What are we going to do with the unrighteousness manifesting through us? Romans 7:19 goes on to say (in my paraphrase), "For the good that I want to do, I do not do it. And the evil that I wish I would not do, that is what I do. Now if I do those things that I wish I would not do, it is no more I that am doing it, but sin that dwelleth in me that is now doing it."

[19]For the good that I would I do not: but
the evil which I would not, that I do.
[20]Now if I do that I would not, it is no
more I that do it, but sin that dwelleth
in me. Romans 7:19-20 KJV

When I have a saint who comes to me oppressed by a devil, or maybe they are filled with various evil spirits, I am able to separate them from that evil. My mindset when dealing with believers who have devils is not to judge them by what manifests. I do not identify people by the evil spirits that are tormenting them. By doing so, I am able to see them as God sees them from the foundation of the world. He intended for us to be perfect and pure, but spiritual entities that have joined us from the fall of Adam and Eve. God did not make creation defective. In fact, He said it was very good, including humanity.

*And God saw every thing that he had
made, and, behold, it was very good.
And the evening and the morning were
the sixth day. Genesis 1:31 KJV*

So, it is not humanity that was created
defective, but the evil that joined us is the defect we
see manifesting every day. That is the sin that dwells
within. This is the evil that must go. When I minister
to people, I help them forgive others because they are
able to separate the sin in that person from the person
themselves. Part of the work of Satan's kingdom is to
convince us we are sin—that it is an inescapable part
of who we are. If someone believes they *are* the evil
manifesting out of them, I cannot cast *them* out of
themselves. However, if I can help them to discern an
evil spirit that has joined their personality, it can be
removed from them, and they may be freed to be
conformed to the image of Christ.

I help people get freedom by helping them
separate themselves from Satan's nature, known as
sin, in their lives. Sometimes we become so entwined
in the way we think, speak, and act with the nature of
Satan in our lives we become one with it. How many
people struggle with a spirit of fear, so they become
one with it? How many of us struggle with self-
hatred so much that we become one with it and we
believe it is us? It is not us; it is the "sin that dwelleth
within" that has become one with us. But sin is not
our identity.

The imperfect aspects of our lives are not part of our identity. So, yes, we are a new creature, but we are leavened by sin, even after the new birth. The evil aspects that manifest out of us are not us. We are not fear, envy, jealousy, divination, bitterness, doubt, unbelief, lust, or any other sins. They are not part of the identity that Father God established for us, but they have become part of our existence. They are hitchhikers and spiritual parasites that have joined themselves to us in our family trees or our personal lives that are part of us on a day-to-day basis. However, does Father God see them as a part of our core identity? No. Do I believe they are part of our identity? No. But, I have to be honest; they did not pass away when we became born again because we are still manifesting them. And they are here today. This is what Paul was dealing with—a great, pragmatic application of the process of sanctification, understanding, and discernment of spiritual things.

APPROPRIATE THE PROMISES

So, yes, I am a new creature, by faith. Yes, I am a new creature and, yes, all the promises of God are yea and amen. Yes, all the promises are mine and by His stripes, I am healed. But I still have to appropriate them, and nobody teaches appropriation these days. Three words in Scripture are still valid to the Christian Church, but nobody teaches them. These words are *if*, *then*, and *but*. We are taught the promises are all ours, unconditionally, without any responsibility on our part to appropriate them out of obedience and sanctification. I do not teach this position on *if*, *then*, and *but* because I just had a thought or a personal revelation. I am a guy who is involved in people's lives, and by becoming involved in people's lives, I have bumped into these issues; therefore, I am stuck dealing with them.

I wish I was not forced to deal with the subject of appropriation. It would be more fun not to have a ministry that deals with appropriation—we would just get people saved. However, I will say that salvation does not begin in the new birth. It begins AFTER the new birth. The new birth is God's grace and mercy for us out of His love. Then comes the process of rebirth. See, we have the new birth, but then we have the *rebirth* afterward, known as sanctification. I am not using the term from the New Age standpoint of rebirth. That is a damaging New Age term. However, according to Scripture, we are being changed.

We are in a state of metamorphosis. How do I know that? Because the Word of God says that we are changed "from glory to glory."

> *But we all, with open face beholding as in a glass the glory of the Lord, are changed into the same image from glory to glory, even as by the Spirit of the Lord. 2 Corinthians 3:18 KJV*

At what point do we begin to be changed into His image? Does it happen at the moment of the new birth or AFTER the new birth? Are we being changed at the new birth, or are we being changed after the new birth? Why do we read our Bibles? Why do we pray about our lives? Why do we do most tasks in our lives? Because we need a change. There is something that needs to be improved in our lives. There are aspects of our lives that need to be cleansed. There are areas of our thought processes that need the renewing of our minds. There are areas of our lives in need of sanctification. There are areas of our lives that need deliverance and healing. There needs to be a cleaning up so that the Church can be presented without spot or blemish.

> *That he might present it to himself a glorious church, not having spot, or wrinkle, or any such thing; but that it should be holy and without blemish. Ephesians 5:27 KJV*

When do we deal with spots and blemishes, at the new birth or after? I will tell you, I have not found a Christian yet who did not have spots and blemishes. They did not go away when we became born again. Now there are some exceptions to this, and I have observed God heal people instantly upon conversion. He has delivered many of them of bondages immediately upon conversion. Many of us have our stories of instant change at the new birth. But, when the honeymoon was over after the new birth experience, many still dealt with the consequences of sin in parts of their lives.

A LIFELONG EXPERIENCE

Now, can we meet each other in love and our own processes of growth? Then we are able to work together and with the Holy Spirit. Sanctification is a lifelong experience, and the basis for our entrance into heaven is not our "sinlessness". Our faith in the Lord Jesus Christ and what He did for us at the cross forms a proper basis. Let us read further in Romans 7:20-21.

> *Now if I do that I would not, it is no more I that do it, but sin that dwelleth in me. Romans 7:20 KJV*

In verse 21, Paul, a Christian and an apostle, is speaking. "I find then a law, that, when I would do good, evil is present with me."

> *I find then a law, that, when I would do good, evil is present with me. Romans 7:21 KJV*

So even though Paul has the law of God, what else is in him? The law of evil. Have any of us ever found ourselves struggling with good and evil? Have we ever found ourselves weighing and considering what was of God and what was not of God? Have we ever considered if we were listening to the devil? Have devils ever come to us and talked to us? Remember, Satan can come as an angel of light.

*And no marvel; for Satan himself is
transformed into an angel of light. 2
Corinthians 11:14 KJV*

We have to watch out for him; he comes as an
angel of light because he wants to be the most high
God. The devil can come and pretend he is God.
Through his kingdom, he can come and say he is
God. He can come saying God is speaking to us
when, in fact, it is Satan. The devil can come and tell
us that he is God and that God is speaking to us.
Have we read that he said he would be like the most
high God?

*[12]How art thou fallen from heaven, O
Lucifer, son of the morning! how art
thou cut down to the ground, which
didst weaken the nations! [13]For thou
hast said in thine heart, I will ascend
into heaven, I will exalt my throne
above the stars of God: I will sit also
upon the mount of the congregation, in
the sides of the north: [14]I will ascend
above the heights of the clouds; I will be
like the most High. [15]Yet thou shalt be
brought down to hell, to the sides of the
pit. Isaiah 14:12-15 KJV*

I believe the devil has the most fun in the
Christian Church. If I were a devil, I would go find a
Christian because that is where I would have fun. The
devil and his kingdom are very spiritual, and they
want to join God's program. They want to be like God

and they do that through divination. A spirit of divination is a counterfeit for the Holy Spirit. Religion is a counterfeit for the Kingdom of God. How does this happen? I have already pointed out many examples where Christianity holds opinions contrary to the Bible. Where did they come from? They are right-sounding religious ideas that put believers into bondage. Is it possible that we are hearing ideas from spirits of divination and parroting them as Scriptural concepts? These ideas are close to the truth. They used to tell me the distance between sanity and insanity was a hair's breadth. Sometimes it is that close. The only sanity we have is what the Word of God says about subjects; this is the only sanity that we have. Let God be true and every man a liar.

> *God forbid: yea, let God be true, but every man a liar; as it is written, That thou mightest be justified in thy sayings, and mightest overcome when thou art judged. Romans 3:4 KJV*

APPLICATION OF TRUTH

Back to Romans 7:21. Paul is saying that when he would do good, evil was present with him.

> *I find then a law, that, when I would do good, evil is present with me. Romans 7:21 KJV*

Moving on to verses 22 and 23, it says, "For I delight in the law of God after the inward man: But I see another law in my members, warring against the law of my mind, and bringing me into captivity to the law of sin which is in my members."

> *[22]For I delight in the law of God after the inward man: [23]But I see another law in my members, warring against the law of my mind, and bringing me into captivity to the law of sin which is in my members. Romans 7:22-23 KJV*

Remember that the law of God is the Word of God. So could I also say he sees another "word" manifesting in his members? This "word" is warring against the Word of God, or the law of his mind, and bringing him into captivity to the law of sin, which was in his members. So, where was the evil? Inside of Paul. Where was the law of God? Also, inside his members. It was not just the fiery dart of temptation. He was dealing with the evil of indwelling sin. One day when I see Paul in Heaven, I will hug him because he set me free through his honesty. I am able to have my true identity straightened out once and for all because he identified our spiritual battle.

Where do most Christians go when they see evil inside themselves? They feel stuck because they have been taught that they cannot have evil. They immediately fall into condemnation, guilt, and oppression because they feel something is wrong with them. They do not feel they are really saved or that God loves them. And that is where they stay until somebody, like myself, comes along and says, "Sin is not you. It is not you. Your heart is not evil, and you serve God after the law of God. But there is sin in your life that is being sanctified."

If we are not careful, we get stuck in an organization or church somewhere that says, "Well, you just need to try harder. You just need to pray more, believe more, and fast more. If you feel condemned by sin, you have just not received who you are. Just start walking in it. You just need to read your Bible more, pray more, walk in it more, and just focus on who you are in Christ."

Just because I am focusing on who I am in Christ, it does not deliver me from evil. It establishes my identity but does not mean I do not need sanctification. Merely knowing the promises of Scripture does not produce deliverance. We may have read or heard the Scripture that says when we know the truth, the truth shall set us free.

And ye shall know the truth, and the truth shall make you free. John 8:32 KJV

But truth, in itself, does not set us free; application of truth makes us free. Scripture also says not to be a hearer only of the Word but a doer also.

But whoso looketh into the perfect law of liberty, and continueth therein, he being not a forgetful hearer, but a doer of the work, this man shall be blessed in his deed. James 1:25 KJV

The Church is filled with knowledge, it stinks to high heaven, and they cannot walk in freedom. Why? Because the Church is pretending it does not have evil. And if someone points out a defect in them, they might reply, "Well, the sin you see in me is just my flesh. That is just my flesh." What are we? Are we a split personality? What do we mean by "our flesh"? Are we a split personality, partially sinful and partially righteous? I am not a split personality. It is not my flesh doing it, it is sin that dwells in me. But Henry, the man, is a son of God by faith. And I know my identity and everything that does not match that identity has to go. And I am not one with sin. I may have sin in my life, but I am not sin. I am one with my Father, which is in heaven. But I will be honest, I also have sin in my life that I deal with every single day. According to Scripture, we are to be one with Christ and the Father. Do we become part of the Godhead? No. However, we do follow the Word of God which points us back to the will of Father God. That is how we become *one* with the Father and the Son.

> [20]*Neither pray I for these alone, but for them also which shall believe on me through their word;* [21]*That they all may be one; as thou, Father, art in me, and I in thee, that they also may be one in us: that the world may believe that thou hast sent me. John 17:20-21 KJV*

SPOTS AND BLEMISHES

Returning to my subject, what I am dealing with today is not as much as I dealt with last year, five years ago, or even ten years ago. I am more sanctified today than I was ten years ago. I am also more sanctified today than I was five years ago, and I will be more sanctified tomorrow than I am today because I am working out my salvation daily.

Maybe people see problems in my life. If they see any spots and blemishes in me, it is imperative to go to Galatians 6:1-2.

> *1Brethren, if a man be overtaken in a fault, ye which are spiritual, restore such an one in the spirit of meekness; considering thyself, lest thou also be tempted. 2Bear ye one another's burdens, and so fulfil the law of Christ. Galatians 6:1-2 KJV*

We have no choice. Can I trust others with my spots and blemishes? Someone may say, "Oh, I do not have any, but I know you do." However, I know they have problems in their lives. That is not esoteric knowledge. It does not take a word of knowledge about their lives to figure it out. If we just spend time around each other for a while, it will show up. And if someone tries to hide it, tell me one disease they have, and I will get an indication of their spirituality because their disease often indicates the spiritual root. But the good news is that I do not judge people after Satan's nature manifesting in their lives. I do not judge them after the sin that dwells within them. I do not judge them after the law that they are following. I judge them after how He saw them from the foundation of the world. This is not a judgment of whether they are doing everything right but a statement of faith according to the Word of God. It is a statement of faith that what the Bible says God designed us to be is who we truly are, even if we are not manifesting it yet.

> *But, beloved, we are persuaded better things of you, and things that accompany salvation, though we thus speak. Hebrews 6:9 KJV*

I am holding out for people that the Holy Spirit will perfect them in their generation. We are to be a shining example of God's power over evil. We have been created to the praise of His glory.

> *[11]In whom also we have obtained an inheritance, being predestinated according to the purpose of him who worketh all things after the counsel of his own will: [12]That we should be to the praise of his glory, who first trusted in Christ. Ephesians 1:11-12 KJV*

AN APOSTLE'S HONESTY ABOUT SIN

Let us move over to verse 24 of Romans 7. It says, "O wretched man that I am!"

> *O wretched man that I am! who shall deliver me from the body of this death? Romans 7:24 KJV*

Paul is the writer; I love his honesty. Are we interested in being ministered to by someone who has issues in their life? Paul described himself as a wretched man and chief of sinners.

O wretched man that I am! who shall deliver me from the body of this death? Romans 7:24 KJV

This is a faithful saying, and worthy of all acceptation, that Christ Jesus came into the world to save sinners; of whom I am chief. 1 Timothy 1:15 KJV

I had someone come here a while ago. I was teaching one day, and I like to challenge people in their thinking. To challenge them, I refer to sin in my life to see how they react to the reality that I am not sinless. I said, "I still have 17 devils that I have not dealt with yet." This particular individual asked, "What am I doing at this ministry? That man just got up and said he had 17 devils, and I came here to be healed. I have come here for my own life and he is demonized." Their statement got back to me, and I approached this individual and said, "I heard about your comment regarding what I said." I went on to say, "If I have 17 devils, how many do you have?" Additionally, I added, "You know, that is not much compared to the 486 I had two years ago."

I was not being literal, but I was making a point. We are looking for "perfect" people to minister to us. However, when we minister to others, it is not because we are sinless that the Holy Spirit works with us. Many people are so afraid of evil that they do not want to face it. We do not have to be afraid of evil. We do not have to be afraid of Satan himself. If someone is afraid of him, they have probably watched too many horror movies. As a result, they have transferred evil into them and fear of evil because they watched and entertained their thoughts and imaginations. God is on the throne; He is greater than the devil. And by the way, Proverbs 26:2 is still true: the curse without a cause does not come.

> *As the bird by wandering, as the swallow by flying, so the curse causeless shall not come. Proverbs 26:2 KJV*

If we want the curse to come, we can open up ourselves to fear about evil, and it is right there. How do we do this? A fearful thought may come to remind us of something evil we may have seen in the past. It then projects that evil conclusion onto our lives. If we are unaware that an evil spirit is tempting us, it is easy to accept this thought and become afraid. This is how fear of evil becomes a part of our lives. We do not have to be afraid of evil.

Now, Paul said, "O wretched man that I am. who shall deliver me from the body of this death? I thank God through Jesus Christ our Lord."

> *[24]O wretched man that I am! who shall deliver me from the body of this death?*

²⁵I thank God through Jesus Christ our Lord. So then with the mind I myself serve the law of God; but with the flesh the law of sin. Romans 7:24-25 KJV

So what does Paul need? Deliverance. Even an apostle, he needed deliverance. Who else might need it today? I need deliverance. Oh, wretched man that I am. I am born again and filled with the Holy Spirit. I have been casting out devils, healing the sick, preaching the Gospel of the Kingdom—but I also have problems in my life and sometimes I get sick. What a wonderful thought. Not that he needed deliverance, but the wonderful part is his authenticity and honesty. Romans 7 is so real to me because it meets the conditions of the everyday life of an everyday believer. It brings these Scriptures down to our daily application and the reality of the spiritual battle going on in our lives. It is healthy and wonderful to be able to discern our enemy, and to look at our sin without running from it and avoiding it in guilt and fear. It removes the power of Satan's kingdom to control and torment us. It is powerful to be able to look at our enemy at that level and not run from him.

We have a buddy in heaven named Paul, and he wrote this to teach us if we will read it. How many people read Romans 7 and understand what he is saying? Referring to this subject, I heard a preacher say, "Oh, yes, but Paul was talking about himself before he was saved, having issues with sin." Except Paul does not say that and we will not find that here.

Because Paul, in the context of having evil, said he delighted in God after the inward man.

> ²²*For I delight in the law of God after the inward man:* ²³*But I see another law in my members, warring against the law of my mind, and bringing me into captivity to the law of sin which is in my members. Romans 7:22-23 KJV*

So he was born again, and this statement was after his revelation. So that opinion does not stand the test of Scripture. Look at what Paul says, "I thank God through Jesus Christ our Lord. So then with the mind I myself serve the law of God; but with the flesh the law of sin."

> *I thank God through Jesus Christ our Lord. So then with the mind I myself serve the law of God; but with the flesh the law of sin. Romans 7:25 KJV*

SIN COMEST TO TEMPT

What does it mean to serve the law of God with our minds but the law of sin with our flesh? The *flesh* is the demonic side of me serving the law of sin or Satan. In the area of forgiveness, using this as an example, we may begin to follow the law of God found in the Scriptures. We decide to forgive our brother because that is just the way we are, as our nature has been renewed by God. We have chosen to forgive "seventy times seven," but then sin comes to tempt us. A root of bitterness begins to spring up because of some offense, and we start holding resentment and unforgiveness. If we do that, we are following the law of sin. Where is the root of bitterness taking hold? Here is a Scripture—Hebrews 12:15 says, "Looking diligently lest any man fail of the grace of God; lest any root of bitterness springing up trouble you, and thereby many be defiled."

> *Looking diligently lest any man fail of the grace of God; lest any root of bitterness springing up trouble you, and thereby many be defiled; Hebrews 12:15 KJV*

Springing up where? Within us. Do we feel it? Is it not amazing how we think about Aunt Sally in our minds, but we feel angry about her around our gut? We feel Aunt Sally in our gut because that is where the evil spirit of unforgiveness is—in the human spirit. As a reminder, our human spirit is around our belly.

> *[38]He that believeth on me, as the scripture hath said, out of his belly shall flow rivers of living water. [39](But this spake he of the Spirit, which they that believe on him should receive: for the Holy Ghost was not yet given; because that Jesus was not yet glorified.) John 7:38-39 KJV*

When unforgiveness and the spirit of Bitterness have been dealt with and cast out from our lives, we may think about Aunt Sally, but we do not feel anything about her in our gut anymore. We just have the memory. She may have treated us very poorly, but we have exchanged bitterness for compassion. Paul taught us the evil in her that made her that way; it was not actually her. Now we do not make her evil anymore; we make the devil evil, and we have compassion on Aunt Sally. We made the great exchange from bitterness to compassion. Is that not what God did for us? He made the great exchange from bitterness to compassion and accepted us when we did not deserve it. But we repented, and He forgave us when we were born again.

WALK AFTER THE SPIRIT

Let us go a little further with this subject. The chapter markers in the Bible are not original to the text. When Paul wrote Romans, he did not create chapter divisions. I believe that chapter 8 should be part of chapter 7 because there is a continuum of thought. In verse 1 of Romans 8, it says, "There is therefore now no condemnation to them which are in Christ Jesus."

There is therefore now no condemnation to them which are in Christ Jesus, who walk not after the flesh, but after the Spirit. Romans 8:1 KJV

Let me stop right here and teach. A few years ago, a Christian brother called me. He was having some difficulties in his life. In fact, they were pretty serious, and his whole family was in jeopardy. There were a lot of problems going on. As a result, he heard about my ministry, and he called me. He attended a church that taught that there is no condemnation whatsoever when someone becomes born again. They teach that people are entirely free — we are a new creation and a new creature. We are totally sinless and free. He was taught that level of freedom, but his personal life was the opposite. And because he had problems in his life with a core spiritual problem and the fruit of it, he called me on the phone from his office.

I listened to him for a few minutes, and I said, "Brother, you have sin in your life." He got very huffy with me and said, "Pastor, let me tell you something. You err." I replied, "Okay, how do I err?" He said, "Have you not heard in Romans 8:1 that 'therefore, there is now no condemnation for those who are in Christ Jesus'?" I said, "Why not read part B of that Scripture?" He said, "There is none." I said, "You have an NIV (New International Version), is that right?" He said, "Yes." Then he asked, "What Bible are you reading?" I said, "I am not reading the minority text that you have. I am reading from the majority text version of the King James." I asked, "Do you want me to read you part B?" In response, he asked, "What does it say?"

I replied, "It says, just like your Bible says, 'There is therefore now no condemnation to them which are in Christ Jesus.' However, in the NIV and all the new translations, they have entirely eliminated the last part of this verse. It does not exist. The full statement in the King James Version continues by saying, 'Who walk not after the flesh, but after the Spirit.' Sir, as a born-again saint, if you walk after Satan and his kingdom, there is condemnation. I do not care if you are born again or not. However, when you walk after the Spirit of God, which is the law of God found in the Word of God, there is no condemnation. But, if you are not walking after the Spirit of God, then you are falling back under that old law of sin that is in your members. The law of sin is those issues in your life for which you have not repented. In those areas, you are condemned."

There is therefore now no condemnation to them which are in Christ Jesus, who walk not after the flesh, but after the Spirit. Romans 8:1 KJV

I do not care if someone is born again or not. The curse shall surely come, and there is no provision of safety for us until we deal with sin. If anyone disagrees with me, what is their answer as to why Christians are sick, demonized, and insane? In response, please do not accuse God, claiming sickness and insanity is His will. I cannot accept such conclusions. Paul set me free and allowed me to have my true identity by separating insanity and sickness from God's will for my life. For a while, when I was younger in the Lord, I saw the evil in my life, and I thought that it was me. People in churches kept telling me I was a new creature and a new creation, and even though I knew this, I still felt evil because I knew I had sin in my life. Knowing we are supposed to be righteous when we still have spiritual issues is torment. It is tormenting when we know we are supposed to have good thoughts and do not have them.

What are we going to do with this conflict? I am a new creature in Christ Jesus. It is true that "old things are passed away; behold, all things are become new."

Therefore if any man be in Christ, he is a new creature: old things are passed away; behold, all things are become new. 2 Corinthians 5:17 KJV

But it is also important that we leave those things that are behind. So, what are we to do instead? Let us press on. Why press on? Because we have a journey ahead of us called the "pilgrim's progress", and day by day, I appropriate the promises of God in my life and my true identity as I know it according to the Bible. However, there are parts of my true identity I am not walking in yet. And I may never walk in them all the way. Nonetheless, I press on to continue to grow every day.

12Not as though I had already attained, either were already perfect: but I follow after, if that I may apprehend that for which also I am apprehended of Christ Jesus. 13Brethren, I count not myself to have apprehended: but this one thing I do, forgetting those things which are

behind, and reaching forth unto those
things which are before, ¹⁴I press toward
the mark for the prize of the high calling
of God in Christ Jesus. Philippians 3:12-
14 KJV

THE RIGHTEOUSNESS OF GOD

To expand on this subject, we need to go to Revelation 19:7.

Let us be glad and rejoice, and give
honour to him: for the marriage of the
Lamb is come, and his wife hath made
herself ready. Revelation 19:7 KJV

This is a wonderful Scripture, and it matches up with 2 Corinthians 7:1 as a harmony of Scripture.

Having therefore these promises, dearly
beloved, let us cleanse ourselves from
all filthiness of the flesh and spirit,
perfecting holiness in the fear of God. 2
Corinthians 7:1 KJV

Revelation 19:7 says, "Let us be glad and rejoice, and give honour to him: for the marriage of the Lamb is come, and his wife hath made herself ready." Moving on to verse 8, it says, "And to her was granted that she should be arrayed in fine linen, clean and white: for the fine linen is the righteousness of the saints."

And to her was granted that she should
be arrayed in fine linen, clean and
white: for the fine linen is the
righteousness of saints. Revelation 19:8
KJV

It is not a literal robe of white we will be
wearing in the future; it is the righteousness of God in
us, and we are currently making ourselves ready for
our husband-to-be. I call it the "Holy Ghost bubble
bath time" or the "Holy Ghost shower time". This
church and ministry have been called a spiritual car
wash. My mission is to get the saints, otherwise
known as the Bride of Christ, ready for her
husband — they need some cleaning up or a "scrub-a-
dub-dub".

When I minister, I care for people's hearts. As
they are getting their "car wash," I will clean their
fenders and around their hub caps. I am going to
make sure I do not scratch them. However, when they
come in with mud all over them, I will look at them
and say, "That mud on you is not you. Because
underneath that mud is a sparkling chrome job. You
are a 'classy chassy.' That is you. That is the REAL
you."

So I am not intimidated by what I see when I
find sin in people's lives. According to Scripture, I see
who they were meant to be from the foundation of the
world. I know their proper identity, but I know they
have been through the blemishes of their generations
and the spots of their lives. They might have spiritual

halitosis that may be leaving debris all over others, and yet God still loves them and wants to care for them even as they learn to overcome it. This is part of why I say our attitude toward sin is so important. We are not perfect, and sometimes as we are seeking to follow God, we have sin manifesting in our lives. If God judged us by performance and sinlessness, we would never be able to grow up because we all begin with sins in our lives we cannot see nor understand. Father God works with our hearts' desires to repent even as we do not see these sins. As we desire to change, the Holy Spirit convicts us of sin so we may repent and resist sin as we grow up spiritually.

God loves us despite sin in our lives, and He is rooting for us to overcome sin, which is the bottom line. Father God wants us to overcome sin in our lives. When reading Revelation 2 and 3, it says, "To him that overcometh" and "He that overcometh". It is evident that the prize belongs to those who overcome — the overcomer.

He that hath an ear, let him hear what the Spirit saith unto the churches; To him that overcometh will I give to eat of the tree of life, which is in the midst of the paradise of God. Revelation 2:7 KJV

He that hath an ear, let him hear what the Spirit saith unto the churches; He that overcometh shall not be hurt of the second death. Revelation 2:11 KJV

*²⁶And he that overcometh, and keepeth
my works unto the end, to him will I
give power over the nations: ²⁷And he
shall rule them with a rod of iron; as the
vessels of a potter shall they be broken
to shivers: even as I received of my
Father. Revelation 2:26-27 KJV*

Someone may say it is a lot of work to
overcome, but I will say it is *wonderful* work. It is
"works of righteousness". I enjoy being in the "car
wash of God". I enjoy the convicting work of the Holy
Spirit, spotlighting the sin in my life that needs to be
removed. Condemnation is of the devil, but
conviction is a wonderful work of the Holy Spirit.
Unfortunately, or maybe fortunately, condemnation
and conviction say the same things. Condemnation
and conviction show us the same things, but one is
the devil oppressing us and telling us that that is our
identity. Conviction tells us what we are being
condemned for is not our identity. Condemnation
comes and lays the problems of our lives on us and
says that is our identity. Conviction comes along and
says, "No, that is not our identity. I want to remove
it." Condemnation makes us one with the evil.
Conviction separates us from it. Condemnation is
oppressive. Conviction is healthy and wonderful, and
I love it when the Lord comes and convicts me.

When I feel condemned in my conviction, it is
evidence of the devil and his kingdom — and I tell
them to go jump in the Lake of Fire. If God is working
with me to overcome certain issues and I am being

accused of not being fully sanctified, I am not listening. And when it feels like too much and the devil comes around and really chews off my ears in the process of sanctification, I finally just put my feet down and say, "Listen, you are not my Father. If I have a spiritual problem, it is my Father God's problem. He loves me, and He is going to work it out of my life. So buzz off, Jack. Buzz off. I am not interested in what you have to say. I have a loving Father who saved me."

The funny thing about their accusations is that God saved me when I was living in 99% darkness and full of sin. Now, I am only 43% darkness, which is evidence Father God has been sanctifying me. Yet, the devil comes along and tells me that I am still not clean when I am not nearly as sinful as when I began this journey. Is it not amazing that we responded to God's love when we were really dirty? But now that we are being cleaned up, we no longer believe God loves us. Why is that? Because the devil comes along to remind us of our spots and blemishes. Well, our spots and blemishes are a reminder of who the devil is, not a reminder of who we truly are. I want to repeat myself for emphasis. The spots and the blemishes are a reminder of who the devil is — not who we are.

THE BRIDE PREPARES HERSELF

We are in the process of being sanctified. Indeed, I am a new creature. I am not what I am going to be, but in the future, I shall be changed in the twinkling of an eye. In the meantime, I am preparing myself for my husband. Father God, thank You for returning me to Jesus. Jesus, I am Your wife-to-be (because the Marriage Supper of the Lamb has not yet happened). I want to continue to be sanctified because it is very good.

I want faith to be quickened in people. I want people to be able to look up past the ceiling with eyes of faith into heaven, and I want them to be able to pray, "Father God, thank You for betrothing me to Jesus. Jesus, You are my husband-to-be, and I will be Your wife forever. I am down here on this planet preparing myself for You. Thank You for working with me, and showing me my true identity according to the Word. I am not a spiritual harlot. I may have been a harlot in my past, but that was because I was lost. But I am so happy that You love me. Amen."

Now, some who are older may remember their past as a young man or woman. When we first began to, as I call it, "sparking" or falling in love — it was amazing. We need to keep this same level of freshness of love going with God all the time. By repenting for sin, the Bride of Christ is preparing herself by taking extra time to clean out the spiritual crevices and other parts that don't align with the Word of God. So when Christ comes to the door, we are prepared for Him.

We want there to be a smile on His face and an expectation of love and fun because we have prepared for His coming. We ought to be preparing for the Lord Jesus now every single minute of our lives so we may enter into that place as His help and wife in the future. While my husband-to-be, Jesus, is in the gates of the city with the elders of the land, I will be the *Proverbs 31 Woman*. I am not a literal female, but I perform the same functions as the *Proverbs 31 Woman* by taking care of the affairs of the house while Jesus is away at the gates. The Bride of Christ is much like the *Proverbs 31 Woman* in that we are working with Jesus in the future.

> *Her husband is known in the gates, when he sitteth among the elders of the land. Proverbs 31:23 KJV*

> *She looketh well to the ways of her household, and eateth not the bread of idleness. Proverbs 31:27 KJV*

Whether we are human males or females, we are part of the Bride of Christ and will be the wife of Christ. If we can bring this dimension and eternal perspective into our personal lives, homes, marriages, and relationships, then the devil will be defeated.

As Kings and Priests in the making, we shall follow the Lamb wherever He goes.

> *And hath made us kings and priests unto God and his Father; to him be glory and dominion for ever and ever. Amen. Revelation 1:6 KJV*

As I conclude this topic, I would like to pray. Father God, thank You for giving us Scripture to address the topic of our identity, even our identity after the new birth. Father, let us understand and be able to bridge between Your promises and the fulfillment of those promises. I have seen evidence that just because we have been given promises in the Bible does not mean that they have been fulfilled in our lives to the degree that You have intended for us. Lifelong, we are appropriating Your goodness and Your righteousness to our lives. Day by day, we are being changed. From glory to glory, we are being changed into Your image.

Father, let the sanctifying work of the Holy Spirit—the fire that purges us of all dross and uncleanness—never be lifted from our hearts. Satan, I choose to subject you and your kingdom to the scrutiny of the living God. Even as people read this, I want them to say this next part out loud if they are willing. Say, "Father, take not thy Holy Spirit from me. Take not the purging fire of the Holy Spirit from my life. And let every principality and power be fully exposed and let the light of the glorious Gospel of Jesus Christ shine on their existence. And let all cleansing of the filthiness of the flesh and the spirit be accomplished in my life. Let conviction come. Let the freedom of God come. Let my identity be fully known. I have not been created evil from the foundation of the world. But, from the foundation of the world, God ordained me to be a son and daughter of the living God, and I take my place right now in the name of Jesus. Amen."

Chapter 5: We Have This Hope

FAITH FOR THE FUTURE

Our identity is defined by what is found in the Bible. Even when we see the parts of our lives that are not perfected, our identity is still ours by faith. That puts the devil right back where he needs to be today, under our feet and scrutiny.

> *Thou shalt tread upon the lion and adder: the young lion and the dragon shalt thou trample under feet. Psalm 91:13 KJV*

Being able to be honest about where we are right now — even in our weaknesses and failings — is liberating. Rather than being beaten up by the devil, it puts his kingdom back in the place where we can exercise dominion over him and his kingdom. May the God of peace bruise Satan under our feet shortly.

> *And the God of peace shall bruise Satan under your feet shortly. The grace of our Lord Jesus Christ be with you. Amen. Romans 16:20 KJV*

According to Scripture, we have been seated in heavenly places with Christ Jesus far above all principalities and powers.

> *⁵Even when we were dead in sins, hath quickened us together with Christ, (by*

grace ye are saved;) ⁶And hath raised us
up together, and made us sit together in
heavenly places in Christ Jesus:
Ephesians 2:5-6 KJV

But Paul brought us to a startling reality check.
As he was seated in heavenly places with Christ Jesus
far above all principalities and powers, he still found
them in his life. Just because God is in our life does
not mean the devil has disappeared. It is time to get
all principalities and powers under our feet. It is time
for the sanctifying work of God to come and purge us
of all dross and spots. I trust people are reading this is
because their hearts are open and hungry for this to
happen. I care for every person deeply, and when I
minister to one person, I take it very seriously. One
day Pastor Donna, my wife, said, "Henry, when you
teach, you teach one person as if you are teaching
thousands."

Every last person is so important. Every single
one is so incredibly valuable, so incredibly important,
and so incredibly well worth saving for His glory. Do
we want to be Jesus' wife for all eternity? We are. We
do not have to worry about it. However, have we
walked in that dimension yet? We are part of the
Bride of Christ, which is a journey by faith. We are
betrothed because the Marriage Supper of the Lamb
has not yet happened. We are betrothed during this
lifetime.

We are married by faith. Why did I say we are
married by faith? It means that we have faith for it in

the future and we are learning to walk in what that represents now when we are only betrothed to Christ. To truly understand what I mean, it is important to remember that faith is hope. Do we hope for something we already have in our possession? Do we have faith for the meal we ate last night? No. "Faith is the substance of things hoped for, the evidence of things not seen."

Now faith is the substance of things hoped for, the evidence of things not seen. Hebrews 11:1 KJV

THE MARRIAGE SUPPER OF THE LAMB

We do not have to have faith for being married to Christ if the Marriage Supper of the Lamb has already happened. We have to have faith for it because it is a *future* event. How do we know we have faith? It is very simple: we have hope. If we have hope that we will be married to Christ one day, we have faith. If we feel hopelessness and believe we will not be married to Him, then we do not have faith. However, I believe better things for us. I trust that even if thoughts of doubt attack us from a spirit of doubt and unbelief, we still have hope for the future.

So, we are not currently married to Christ because the event has yet to happen. We are currently betrothed because the Marriage Supper of the Lamb is in the future. There is a great wedding day coming in heaven, and it is not in the carnal sense that we would think of a husband and wife on earth today. It is not carnal making this unclean whatsoever. It is not sexual in the earthly sense but in the mystical sense of union of heart and purpose. We will follow Christ in ruling over this planet with Him. The wife of Him is who we are. If we could get this into our hearts and solidify it, we could never be ripped off by the devil again. Do we believe we will be the wife of Christ for eternity? If so, do not ever let it go. I will practice being a good wife-to-be to Jesus now, not waiting until I get to heaven. I am going to be His wife, and I am going to practice being His wife now, not just after the Marriage Supper of the Lamb.

When I get to the Marriage Supper, that marriage in heaven is going to be incredibly meaningful to me. Let us read from Revelation 19 again. Verse 7 begins, "Let us be glad and rejoice, and give honour to him: for the marriage of the Lamb is come." Now, this is not present progressive. This is prophetic conclusion, but it has not yet happened. Continuing, "For the marriage of the Lamb is come, and his wife hath made herself ready." Hallelujah!

> *Let us be glad and rejoice, and give honour to him: for the marriage of the Lamb is come, and his wife hath made herself ready. Revelation 19:7 KJV*

THE MILLENNIAL REIGN

What if we do not prepare ourselves to rule and reign with Christ, as His wife, in the future? I can see the Lord asking us one day in His millennial reign, "I want you to go over to a certain foreign country to deal with a dictator over there." And we say to him, "Lord, I am too afraid." What do we have to be delivered from in our life? Fear. That is just a crude example of the importance of preparing ourselves today. Fear of man is a serious spiritual issue. The spirit of fear of man is a significant problem for many people. How many of us struggle with fear of man? We cannot witness to people on the street because somebody might look cross-eyed at us, let alone deal with a dictator in a foreign land. I can see us going over to one of these countries and saying to a dictator, "I want to see you in church this Sabbath," and he says, "Go jump in the lake." And we put out tails between our legs and say, "Lord, the dictator said to go jump in the lake. I cannot handle it."

I can also see one of us going over to Hollywood, and the Lord says to one of us, "Go win one of the famous actors or actresses to the Lord." And this person starts to lust after us. What we going to do? Are we going to be like one of those angels who sinned, left their proper state of habitation, and lusted after the daughters of men like in Genesis 6? It is my position that these "sons of God" are not humans but angels like the "sons of God" who presented themselves to God in Job.

> *Now there was a day when the sons of God came to present themselves before the LORD, and Satan came also among them. Job 1:6 KJV*

So will we be like one of those beings who chose to rebel against God because of lust?

That the sons of God saw the daughters of men that they were fair; and they took them wives of all which they chose. Genesis 6:2 KJV

There were giants in the earth in those days; and also after that, when the sons of God came in unto the daughters of men, and they bare children to them, the same became mighty men which were of old, men of renown. Genesis 6:4 KJV

Now is time to give up these sins. Give up lust. Give up fear. These are the sins that torment and tempt us, are they not? I love people, and that is why I am confronting this subject. I am not trying to condemn people for sin. But if we struggle with these issues, it is time to cry out to Father God, repent, and learn to resist these evil spirits that will make us unfit to rule and reign with Christ in the future.

THE THIRD HEAVEN

These evil spirits need us because without us they are caught in a place called the second heaven or, as the Bible specifically calls it, the "dry place," as I mentioned previously. It is not in the first heaven where we exist physically. Who is in the third heaven? Father God. Some people attempt to prove and teach seven heavens. That is an occultic idea that occludes or hides the reality described in Scripture. It is an idea coming out of astrology and Eastern Mysticism. In the Bible, there are only three heavens.

Where was Paul caught up to? Into the third heaven.

I knew a man in Christ above fourteen years ago, (whether in the body, I cannot tell; or whether out of the body, I cannot tell: God knoweth;) such an one caught up to the third heaven. 2 Corinthians 12:2 KJV

It was the third heaven, so there must logically also be a first heaven and a second heaven. When we study Scripture, what is the first heaven? As we taught earlier, it is right here in the physical dimension. It is the atmosphere, seven million stars, and the planet Earth on which we live. If there is a first heaven and a third heaven, there must be a second heaven. I am reminding everyone of these principles because Satan is called the prince of the power of the air.

Wherein in time past ye walked according to the course of this world, according to the prince of the power of the air, the spirit that now worketh in the children of disobedience: Ephesians 2:2 KJV

JUDGMENT FOR THE PLANET

He is bound to this planet in judgment, along with every principality, fallen angel, and devil who fell with him. It is my position that Satan was on this planet before Adam and Eve were created when he was known as Lucifer. According to Jeremiah 4, this planet was inhabited before Adam and Eve. In the Spirit World Realities teaching, we have taught this subject in detail. To summarize an essential part of that teaching that is relevant to this subject, I want to connect Genesis 1 and Jeremiah 4. Genesis 1:2 says that the earth was without form and void. Some may argue that it was just in an unformed state, but the Hebrew terms used in this Scripture refer to something that is destroyed and ruined.

> *And the earth was without form, and void; and darkness was upon the face of the deep. And the Spirit of God moved upon the face of the waters. Genesis 1:2 KJV*

I cannot see how Father God would intentionally create something that was in a ruined state when, after creation, He refers to creation as "very good."

> *And God saw every thing that he had made, and, behold, it was very good. And the evening and the morning were the sixth day. Genesis 1:31 KJV*

Beginning in Jeremiah 4:19, it expands upon the events leading up to Genesis 1:2. Jeremiah 4:19-22 details a judgment that occurred on the planet because there was no knowledge of good. They were only wise to do evil.

> *19My bowels, my bowels! I am pained at my very heart; my heart maketh a noise in me; I cannot hold my peace, because thou hast heard, O my soul, the sound of the trumpet, the alarm of war. 20Destruction upon destruction is cried; for the whole land is spoiled: suddenly are my tents spoiled, and my curtains in a moment. 21How long shall I see the standard, and hear the sound of the trumpet? 22For my people is foolish, they have not known me; they are sottish children, and they have none understanding: they are wise to do evil, but to do good they have no knowledge. Jeremiah 4:19-22 KJV*

Jeremiah 4:23-26 describes the earth without form and void and echoes the same phrases from Genesis 1:2. It then details the cities being broken down at the fierce anger of the Lord. It was a warning to the people of Jeremiah's time that judgment had come before, and similar consequences awaited them if they rebelled against God in the present time.

> *23I beheld the earth, and, lo, it was without form, and void; and the heavens, and they had no light. 24I beheld the mountains, and, lo, they trembled, and all the hills moved*

lightly. ²⁵I beheld, and, lo, there was no man, and all the birds of the heavens were fled. ²⁶I beheld, and, lo, the fruitful place was a wilderness, and all the cities thereof were broken down at the presence of the LORD, and by his fierce anger. Jeremiah 4:23-26 KJV

I do not want to distract from this teaching by going into depth on this subject. If anyone is interested in all the proofs, I invite them to invest in my teaching on Spirit World Realities. It is my position from Scripture that this time was ruled by angels—this also included a covering cherub known as Lucifer or *Helel*, translated from the Hebrew. All the kingdoms of that time before Adam and Eve and the beings who lived during that time were judged for their rebellion against God.

I believe they were judged and they became disembodied as a result. In this present time, when we die, where does our body go? Back to the ground and to the dust. But where does our spirit go? Back to God, who gave it.

Then shall the dust return to the earth as it was: and the spirit shall return unto God who gave it. Ecclesiastes 12:7 KJV

Ecclesiastes says that when an animal dies, its spirit goes down into the dust, but the man's spirit goes back to God who gave it.

*Who knoweth the spirit of man that
goeth upward, and the spirit of the
beast that goeth downward to the
earth? Ecclesiastes 3:21 KJV*

But how is our soul retained after we die? Our soul or brain is a part of our physical body. Our soul is a part of our brain cells, but our brain cells die with our body. So how is our soul saved? It is my position that it is preserved because our spirit is eternal. The best I can gather is there is a mirror, or "carbon copy," of our physical existence that is etched into our existence as a human spirit. Therefore, if our soul is saved, our spirit is also saved. If our soul is not saved, our spirit is lost to creation forever.

THE FIRST RESURRECTION

So from this standpoint, can we ever be disembodied and still exist? Where do people go when they die? Heaven or hell. The rich man was conscious in hell, but his body was in the dust.

*22And it came to pass, that the beggar
died, and was carried by the angels into
Abraham's bosom: the rich man also
died, and was buried; 23And in hell he
lift up his eyes, being in torments, and
seeth Abraham afar off, and Lazarus in
his bosom. Luke 16:22-23 KJV*

Lazarus was conscious in the bosom of Abraham after death. Where was he? In paradise. Where was his body? Dust in the earth. Everybody who is in heaven today, Old and New Testament, died in faith. Where are their bodies? Dust in the earth. What are they awaiting in heaven? The First Resurrection. Currently, they are in heaven—the third heaven awaiting the First Resurrection.

> *Blessed and holy is he that hath part in the first resurrection: on such the second death hath no power, but they shall be priests of God and of Christ, and shall reign with him a thousand years. Revelation 20:6 KJV*

All the unrighteous, when they die, where are there bodies? In the ground. And where are their spirits? In hell. They are waiting to be resurrected after the 1000-year reign of Christ for the White Throne Judgment.

> *But the rest of the dead lived not again until the thousand years were finished. This is the first resurrection. Revelation 20:5 KJV*

> *[11]And I saw a great white throne, and him that sat on it, from whose face the earth and the heaven fled away; and there was found no place for them. [12]And I saw the dead, small and great, stand before God; and the books were opened: and another book was opened,*

which is the book of life: and the dead were judged out of those things which were written in the books, according to their works. Revelation 20:11-12 KJV

This is a basic Scriptural teaching. It is a standard, straight-ahead understanding of Scripture about the end of this age. So when we die, will we continue to exist? Yes. But, we will be disembodied. What happened to the beings who lived on this planet who were judged with Lucifer, including the third of the angels who rebelled with him? It is my position that they were all judged and became disembodied. I believe they are the ones caught in the second heaven or "dry place" surrounding this planet.

DISEMBODIED SPIRITS

When Adam and Eve were in the garden, where was Satan? Right there. Was he visible to them in the garden? No. Did Eve see Satan personally? No. So what did he use to manifest himself to Eve? He used a serpent as a medium of expression. After Satan convinced Adam and Eve to sin by eating of the tree they were forbidden to eat from, what came into them? Was it Satan himself? No, other evil spirits that were invisible entered them. What was the first one that came? A spirit of fear. They became afraid of God after they ate the fruit. Then what else came into them? A spirit of shame. After being afraid, they hid from God because they were ashamed that they were naked. The other spirit that entered them was guilt. How do I know guilt entered Adam and Eve? They blamed others rather than taking responsibility for sinning against God.

8And they heard the voice of the LORD God walking in the garden in the cool of the day: and Adam and his wife hid themselves from the presence of the LORD God amongst the trees of the garden. 9And the LORD God called unto Adam, and said unto him, Where art thou? 10And he said, I heard thy voice in the garden, and I was afraid, because I was naked; and I hid myself. 11And he said, Who told thee that thou wast naked? Hast thou eaten of the tree, whereof I commanded thee that thou shouldest not eat? 12And the man said, The woman whom thou gavest to be with me, she gave me of the tree, and I did eat. 13And the LORD God said unto the woman, What is this that thou hast done? And the woman said, The serpent beguiled me, and I did eat. Genesis 3:8-13 KJV

And these spirits came flooding into creation through one man — Adam. Some people state that sin came into the world through Eve, but it was only after Adam ate of the fruit that their eyes were opened, and they saw they were naked.

6And when the woman saw that the tree was good for food, and that it was pleasant to the eyes, and a tree to be

*desired to make one wise, she took of
the fruit thereof, and did eat, and gave
also unto her husband with her; and he
did eat. ⁷And the eyes of them both were
opened, and they knew that they were
naked; and they sewed fig leaves
together, and made themselves aprons.
Genesis 3:6-7 KJV*

Romans states that through one man, sin
entered into the world.

*Wherefore, as by one man sin entered
into the world, and death by sin; and so
death passed upon all men, for that all
have sinned: Romans 5:12 KJV*

If sin entered the world through one man,
would it not already have existed before that
moment? Therefore, it must have existed before it
entered into the world. So, if through one man sin
entered into the world, it already existed in some
form. It is my position, based upon Scriptures, that it
must have been invisible beings we know as evil
spirits today. I consider fear to be a being. I consider
jealousy to be a being. Why do I feel that way? Well,
Numbers mentions jealousy as a spirit.

*And the spirit of jealousy come upon
him, and he be jealous of his wife, and
she be defiled: or if the spirit of jealousy
come upon him, and he be jealous of his
wife, and she be not defiled: Numbers
5:14 KJV*

Or when the spirit of jealousy cometh upon him, and he be jealous over his wife, and shall set the woman before the LORD, and the priest shall execute upon her all this law. Numbers 5:30 KJV

In 2 Timothy, it says that fear is a spirit.

For God hath not given us the spirit of fear; but of power, and of love, and of a sound mind. 2 Timothy 1:7 KJV

In Luke, it says infirmity is a spirit.

And, behold, there was a woman which had a spirit of infirmity eighteen years, and was bowed together, and could in no wise lift up herself. Luke 13:11 KJV

How can the medical community get an evil spirit of infirmity out of a person if they do not cast it out? It is not possible because they do not believe in it. So they have been tricked, and we have been too. I am writing this because I want people to be able to separate themselves from that kingdom, even in disease. It talks, is intelligent, thinks, speaks, has access to us through our spirit, can put thoughts in our head, and can speak to us as if it were God himself. In fact, Satan comes to us through his kingdom as an angel of light.

And no marvel; for Satan himself is transformed into an angel of light. 2 Corinthians 11:14 KJV

But does Satan inhabit us personally? No. So, what is left to represent him? Principalities, powers, rulers of the darkness of this world, and spiritual wickedness in high places — all invisibly influencing us in the second heaven.

For we wrestle not against flesh and blood, but against principalities, against powers, against the rulers of the darkness of this world, against spiritual wickedness in high places. Ephesians 6:12 KJV

Do they have access to human beings? Yes. Can they take over us against our will? No. Can we give place to the devil in our life through sin and temptation? Yes. Do we become one with his nature when we do that? Yes. If it were not the case, we would not have a ministry. It would not be necessary to have a ministry here at all. We would live in a Utopian existence, clapping our hands and singing glory. We can still do that anytime, but I also want everyone to be free. I do not teach just to give some theology or a theory. Knowledge puffeth up and is vanity.

Now as touching things offered unto idols, we know that we all have knowledge. Knowledge puffeth up, but charity edifieth. 1 Corinthians 8:1 KJV

THE FIVE-FOLD MINISTRY

I can teach on a lot of different topics. I have an excellent background in teaching on many subjects. But I am not here to impress anyone or give just some random knowledge. I am here to change lives. I am here to change people's direction. I am here to change people and move them from the kingdom of darkness into the Kingdom of Light. Someone may say, "But I already am in the Kingdom of Light. I am born again." But if someone is in the Kingdom of Light and is born again, why do I see so much darkness manifesting in their life? Why do I see darkness hovering over them in their countenance? I do not see many demons fleeing from their presence. Wherever they walk, I ought to hear demons screaming out of people, "We know who you are, son of God. You have come to torment us before our time." This is what happened to Jesus.

> *²⁸And when he was come to the other side into the country of the Gergesenes, there met him two possessed with devils, coming out of the tombs, exceeding fierce, so that no man might pass by that way. ²⁹And, behold, they cried out, saying, What have we to do with thee, Jesus, thou Son of God? art thou come hither to torment us before the time? Matthew 8:28-29 KJV*

I am in ministry, and I am also teaching others how to minister. I once had about five or six disciples I was teaching. We had just finished a church service, and people would come up to them with all kinds of problems, and I was just supervising. This is the direction for the future. In many parts of Christianity, there is a focus on one person doing all the work of the ministry. Some people are looking for a "spiritual superstar". There is only One and He is in Heaven at the right hand of the Father — Jesus.

Instead, I want to bring the people and teach them to how to handle other people's lives. I want to let the people learn how to take care of the work of the ministry. That is my goal. It is not the five-fold elder's job to be the healers and deliverers, but they have to be here to set the example and set the standard so the sheep can learn. However, the sheep or regular believers should care for other sheep. That is what I read in 1 Corinthians 12. The five-fold elders are there to demonstrate it, oversee it, and ensure it stays in balance. The prophet, the evangelist, the pastor, the apostle, and the teacher ensure that we have the completeness of the Body working together. That is proper Biblical leadership set in place.

> *24For our comely parts have no need: but God hath tempered the body together, having given more abundant honour to that part which lacked: 25That there should be no schism in the body; but that the members should have the same care one for another. 26And whether one member suffer, all the members suffer*

*with it; or one member be honoured, all
the members rejoice with it. ²⁷Now ye
are the body of Christ, and members in
particular. ²⁸And God hath set some in
the church, first apostles, secondarily
prophets, thirdly teachers, after that
miracles, then gifts of healings, helps,
governments, diversities of tongues. 1
Corinthians 12:24-26 KJV*

But the leadership is more fragmented today
than the sheep, both doctrinally and positionally. It is
a mess. The Church is a mess. They may say, "Well,
we are going to heaven." However, between here on
earth and heaven, we have a mess. In the Lord's
Prayer, what does it say? Thy will be done on earth as
it is in heaven. That prayer is an earthly prayer. We
will not be praying that prayer in heaven. When we
get to heaven, we will not need to pray at all. There
will be no reason for us to pray because we will be
right there in the presence of God Himself. Remember
when the Pharisees came to Jesus and asked why His
disciples did not fast and pray like John the Baptist's
disciples did? Jesus told them His disciples did not
have to fast and pray because the *reason* for fasting
and praying was there in their midst. But He said
when He was gone, they should fast and pray
because He would not be there.

*¹⁸And the disciples of John and of the
Pharisees used to fast: and they come
and say unto him, Why do the disciples
of John and of the Pharisees fast, but
thy disciples fast not? ¹⁹And Jesus said*

unto them, Can the children of the
bridechamber fast, while the bridegroom
is with them? as long as they have the
bridegroom with them, they cannot fast.
²⁰But the days will come, when the
bridegroom shall be taken away from
them, and then shall they fast in those
days. Mark 2:18-20 KJV

If that is how it was on earth when the Lord was here, fasting and praying will not be necessary in heaven because we will also be in His presence.

LIGHT DISPELS DARKNESS

Now, before moving on from our subject on separating ourselves from the kingdom of darkness that rules with us, I want to address a question that some people may have challenging my conclusions. Many people reason that because light dispels darkness, we cannot have darkness in our lives if we also have light in our lives. Many people argue this point because they say light and darkness cannot cohabit together. The problem with their reasoning is the assumption that the presence of light automatically dispels darkness. No, light dispels darkness in the context of the spiritual confrontation, but we cannot have a confrontation if we do not bring light and darkness together. If we put light in one room and darkness in another room, we have no change. Therefore, light has to make contact with darkness to have change.

In the room I am in, there is light. But is this room fully filled with light? No. There are shadows and even dark shadows. In Jungian psychology, the things that reside in the "collective subconscious" are called the dark shadows and archetypes. In the Bible, those "archetypes and dark shadows" are called evil spirits, principalities, powers, spiritual wickedness in high places, and rulers of the darkness of this world. Most of the time we are "shadowboxing" our enemy because we do not actually discern their true nature and intent in our lives.

> *For we wrestle not against flesh and blood, but against principalities, against powers, against the rulers of the darkness of this world, against spiritual wickedness in high places. Ephesians 6:12 KJV*

Chapter 6: From Glory to Glory

THE RIGHTEOUSNESS OF THE SAINTS

This brings us to the subject of sanctification. I will be quoting from 2 Corinthians 7:1. It begins by talking about promises; these are the promises that produce sanctification, and they are for the Bride of Christ.

> *Having therefore these promises, dearly beloved, let us cleanse ourselves from all filthiness of the flesh and spirit, perfecting holiness in the fear of God. 2 Corinthians 7:1 KJV*

Remember the passages we read from Revelation 19? Verse 7 begins: "Let us be glad and rejoice, and give honour to him: for the marriage of the Lamb is come, and his wife hath made herself ready."

> *Let us be glad and rejoice, and give honour to him: for the marriage of the Lamb is come, and his wife hath made herself ready. Revelation 19:7 KJV*

Verse 8 continues: "And to her was granted that she should be arrayed in fine linen, clean and white." People often paint pictures of the saints dressed in white. Some have taught it is a garment we will wear. I have heard people talk about wanting to be dressed in a white robe. However, let us consider what the white robe represents. "For the fine linen is the righteousness of saints."

And to her was granted that she should be arrayed in fine linen, clean and white: for the fine linen is the righteousness of saints. Revelation 19:8 KJV

What is the righteousness of the saints? "The kingdom of God is not meat and drink; but righteousness, and peace, and joy in the Holy Ghost."

For the kingdom of God is not meat and drink; but righteousness, and peace, and joy in the Holy Ghost. Romans 14:17 KJV

Righteousness, peace, and joy in the Holy Ghost is the righteousness of the saints. It is not the result of self-righteousness, but the process of repentance and making choices to follow God instead of sin, that changes our lives. Another related part of this topic is the glory of God as the righteousness of God in us. Do we know what the glory of God is? It is not a halo around Jesus' head; the glory of God is God's nature.

The nature of God can be found in the fruits of the Holy Spirit, as seen in Galatians 5.

[22]But the fruit of the Spirit is love, joy, peace, longsuffering, gentleness, goodness, faith, [23]Meekness,

temperance: against such there is no
law. Galatians 5:22-23 KJV

CREATED IN HIS IMAGE

We were created to be formed into His image. In Genesis 1:26, Elohim says, "Let us," this is a plural term because it refers to the Godhead. There are three members of the Godhead — Father God, Jesus/God the Word, and the Holy Spirit. As translated from Hebrew, this would be the *echad* or unity. As I have noted, unity does not consist of a singular entity, so there is our *plural unity* or Godhead. It goes on to say, "Let us make man in our image."

> *And God said, Let us make man in our*
> *image, after our likeness: and let them*
> *have dominion over the fish of the sea,*
> *and over the fowl of the air, and over*
> *the cattle, and over all the earth, and*
> *over every creeping thing that creepeth*
> *upon the earth. Genesis 1:26 KJV*

In other words, if we replace the term God with the English phonetic translation of the Hebrew text, this Scripture begins with *Elohim*. By adding in this term, Genesis 1:26 reads, "And Elohim said, Let us (God the Word, Adonai/Father God, and Holy Spirit) make man in our image." Another way of phrasing it is: "Elohim/God the Word said, Father, let us make man in our image."

How are we created in His image? The first aspect is our human spirit, and how we think. Because as a man thinks in his heart, so is he.

For as he thinketh in his heart, so is he: Eat and drink, saith he to thee; but his heart is not with thee. Proverbs 23:7 KJV

THAT WHICH COMES OUT

Continuing on this subject of the human spirit let us look at Mark 7. The Pharisees had just challenged Jesus about His disciples because they did not wash their hands before eating dinner. How often have we told our kids to wash their hands before dinner?

So Jesus is dealing with this subject to help them understand a deeper spiritual principle, and He says in verse 15: "There is nothing from without a man, that entering into him can defile him: but the things which come out of him, those are they that defile the man. If any man have ears to hear, let him hear. And when he was entered into the house from the people, his disciples asked him concerning the parable. And he saith unto them, Are ye so without understanding also? Do ye not perceive that whatsoever thing from without entereth into the man, it cannot defile him; Because it entereth not into his heart, but into the belly and," — my insertion — goes out into Charmin Land "purging all meats." Of course, I am joking in my phrasing, but we need to stop being so serious.

> *[15]There is nothing from without a man, that entering into him can defile him: but the things which come out of him, those are they that defile the man. [16]If any man have ears to hear, let him hear. [17]And when he was entered into the house from the people, his disciples asked him concerning the parable. [18]And he saith unto them, Are ye so without understanding also? Do ye not perceive, that whatsoever thing from without entereth into the man, it cannot defile him; [19]Because it entereth not into his heart, but into the belly, and goeth out into the draught, purging all meats? Mark 7:15-19 KJV*

And then He said, "That which cometh out of the man, that defileth the man. For from within," I do not mean to stop mid-sentence, but let us consider the word Jesus uses here. "For from within" means that it is inside of us, not external to us. Those things inside of us that manifest through us as sin are those things that truly defile us — not forgetting to wash our hands.

> *[20]And he said, That which cometh out of the man, that defileth the man. [21]For from within, out of the heart of men, proceed evil thoughts, adulteries, fornications, murders, [22]Thefts, covetousness, wickedness, deceit,*

*lasciviousness, an evil eye, blasphemy,
pride, foolishness:* ²³*All these evil things
come from within, and defile the man.*
Mark 7:20-23 KJV

When we read from Romans 7, where did Paul
say sin dwelt? Was sin dwelling outside of him? No.
It dwelt within him. Paul had sin; he said he had sin
twice.

¹⁵*For that which I do I allow not: for
what I would, that do I not; but what I
hate, that do I.* ¹⁶*If then I do that which
I would not, I consent unto the law that
it is good.* ¹⁷*Now then it is no more I
that do it, but sin that dwelleth in me.*
Romans 7:15-17 KJV

And that sin dwelt where? In his flesh.

*For I know that in me (that is, in my
flesh,) dwelleth no good thing: for to
will is present with me; but how to
perform that which is good I find not.*
Romans 7:18 KJV

WASHING OF THE WATER OF THE WORD

The *flesh* of Paul were the evil spirits, and they
dwelt within him. Two main aspects that comprise
the *flesh* are mentioned in this Scripture. Number one,
the flesh are the evil spirits themselves. Number two,

it can also be our minds that have become one with how the spirits programmed us by their nature. If we follow temptation and sin long enough, we begin to think like these evil spirits. We have two dimensions of the flesh. Once the evil spirit is repented of and cast out, we must still undergo the renewing of our minds. The old nature, or the old man, involves our way of thinking that contradicts the Word of God. That is why our mind is renewed by the washing of the water of the Word. The Word of God needs to confront ways of thinking and behaving that represent sin instead of God.

> *[25]Husbands, love your wives, even as Christ also loved the church, and gave himself for it; [26]That he might sanctify and cleanse it with the washing of water by the word, [27]That he might present it to himself a glorious church, not having spot, or wrinkle, or any such thing; but that it should be holy and without blemish. Ephesians 5:25-27 KJV*

However, we cannot stop with the soul because we also have a spirit. It says in the Bible, "Having therefore these promises, dearly beloved, let us cleanse ourselves from all filthiness of the flesh and the spirit."

> *Having therefore these promises, dearly beloved, let us cleanse ourselves from all filthiness of the flesh and spirit, perfecting holiness in the fear of God. 2 Corinthians 7:1 KJV*

So where do we need to be cleansed? Not just in our minds but in our spirits. Someone may say, "But I am born again." Then go up heaven and ask Paul what he meant. That person's argument is not with me; I did not write the Bible. I can only quote and teach it. Paul recognizes that there is another dimension that needs to be cleansed — not just the flesh, not just the soul, but also the human spirit. Remember I quoted from 1 Thessalonians 5:23, which talks about the God of peace sanctifying us wholly? The key emphasis is the spell of that word: w-h-o-l-l-y in spirit, soul, and body.

And the very God of peace sanctify you wholly; and I pray God your whole spirit and soul and body be preserved blameless unto the coming of our Lord Jesus Christ. 1 Thessalonians 5:23 KJV

Hebrews 4:12 says, "For the word of God is quick, and powerful, and sharper than any twoedged sword." It says it is able to penetrate even to the joint and marrow, is a discerner of the thoughts and intents of the heart, and is able to separate the soul from the spirit.

For the word of God is quick, and powerful, and sharper than any twoedged sword, piercing even to the dividing asunder of soul and spirit, and of the joints and marrow, and is a discerner of the thoughts and intents of the heart. Hebrews 4:12 KJV

Right there, we see the Word of God can separate the soul from the spirit. Why would the Word of God be necessary to separate the soul from the spirit? Because the soul and the spirit had become one with the thought processes of the mind of Satan. Now, the Word of God comes and convicts by the Spirit of God to penetrate our human spirit. By the Spirit of God, the Word of God is established in our hearts by truth. As we repent and our minds are continually washed, our way of thinking now becomes one with God in spirit and soul. In the places where we were one with Satan and his kingdom in our thinking, we are now one with God and His way of thinking and His Kingdom instead.

BE A DOER OF THE WORD

In the areas where we have been sanctified by God, that righteousness has become part of our nature—providing we are not just a hearer of the word, but a doer as well. If we have decided in our hearts that we must forgive our brother regardless of what he has done to us, what do we do when our brother offends us? By choosing to forgive, which is God's nature, it becomes righteousness in our lives, which is His glory in us. God's glory in us is not how many miracles we can do. God's glory in us is not if we can heal the sick. God's glory in us is not how many chandeliers we can swing off in a hyped-up religious environment.

God's glory in us is His nature manifested in us as a way of life. Who we are, in the choices we make, reflects His nature according to the Word of God. Essentially, the way we are is the way He is. And together, we are one in thought, deed, and action. Remember the Scripture that says we are changed "from glory to glory"?

But we all, with open face beholding as in a glass the glory of the Lord, are changed into the same image from glory to glory, even as by the Spirit of the Lord. 2 Corinthians 3:18 KJV

What does "from glory to glory" we are being changed mean? From unrighteousness to righteousness, we are being changed. From unforgiveness back over to forgiveness, we are being changed. Is unforgiveness the "glory of God," or is forgiveness the "glory of God"? Is fear the "glory of God," or is faith the "glory of God"? The glory of God is manifested through us as we choose to follow Father God instead of Satan's kingdom. So if we have faith and we have forgiveness as part of the makeup of our character on the inside, then that is His glory manifested in us. We have been raised up and created by Him—to the praise of His glory.

[11]In whom also we have obtained an inheritance, being predestinated according to the purpose of him who worketh all things after the counsel of his own will: [12]That we should be to the

praise of his glory, who first trusted in
Christ. Ephesians 1:11-12 KJV

What is the praise of His glory? When I forgive
my neighbor, I demonstrate the very nature of the
living God on the earth in the midst of unforgiveness.
I also demonstrate it as an aspect of correct spiritual
existence; against that, no law can defeat or bind me.

> [22]*But the fruit of the Spirit is love, joy,*
> *peace, longsuffering, gentleness,*
> *goodness, faith,* [23]*Meekness,*
> *temperance: against such there is no*
> *law. Galatians 5:22-23 KJV*

When I operate according to the nature of the
living God, there is no spiritual foothold Satan's
kingdom can gain in that area of my life. This is not
from legalistically following rules, but because I have
chosen to follow God because it is the best direction
for my life. I have chosen to make it my nature to
forgive. It is my nature to believe. It is my nature to
love. It is my nature to have longsuffering. It is my
nature to be a man of peace. That is in the Psalms. "I
am for peace: but when I speak, they are for war."

> *I am for peace: but when I speak, they*
> *are for war. Psalm 120:7 KJV*

I am a warrior. We are called to be warriors,
not wimpy losers. I love destroying the works of the
devil. I love being anointed by God, and I love
healing all those who are oppressed of the devil. I
love executing authority over a dark kingdom.

OBEDIENCE FULFILLED

There are two aspects to this journey of sanctification that require our attention. We often try to do spiritual warfare and defeat the enemy, but our obedience has not first been fulfilled first. That is why the church is such a miserable failure in defeating disease, insanity, and spiritual problems. We see the promises of God found in the Bible, and we try to execute the Kingdom of God, but our hearts are corrupt because of personal sin. Do we understand that this is a problem? Second Corinthians 10:5 says we should hold every thought in captivity and cast down every imagination, everything that would exalt itself against the knowledge of God."

Casting down imaginations, and every high thing that exalteth itself against the knowledge of God, and bringing into captivity every thought to the obedience of Christ; 2 Corinthians 10:5 KJV

We attempt to apply this verse, but do we quote verse 6 as well? Nobody quotes verse 6, which says, "And having in a readiness to revenge all disobedience, when your obedience is fulfilled."

And having in a readiness to revenge all disobedience, when your obedience is fulfilled. 2 Corinthians 10:6 KJV

Going to Hebrews 4:12, it talks about the Word of God being quick and powerful, sharper than a two-edged sword.

> *For the word of God is quick, and powerful, and sharper than any twoedged sword, piercing even to the dividing asunder of soul and spirit, and of the joints and marrow, and is a discerner of the thoughts and intents of the heart. Hebrews 4:12 KJV*

We all quote that verse, and yes, we need the Word of God. But why do many people fail to quote verse 13? Now, read this carefully: "Neither is there any creature that is not manifest in his sight."

> *Neither is there any creature that is not manifest in his sight: but all things are naked and opened unto the eyes of him with whom we have to do. Hebrews 4:13 KJV*

The Word of God comes to shine a flashlight on the roaches and spiritual parasites of our lives. I consider every evil spirit, principality, and power to be spiritual parasites that suck the life right out of us. Instead of the Holy Spirit influencing our decisions, they speak to us and push us around through temptation. They come in and suck the life out of us and then take our dead, lifeless, incorrect spirituality and existence and raise us back up to the glory of Satan.

They inhabit and rule us, and we become a medium of expression for Satan in the earth. When we hate our brother, we are a medium of expression for hell. When we are full of envy and jealousy, hatred, variance and strife, and every other sin, we are a declaration and an oracle of Satan on the earth by the influence of his kingdom. That is our sin, and we need to repent. Someone may say, "Pastor Henry, you are getting awfully stern." Listen, lives are at stake. Should I teach the truth or teach a lie? I am working out my own salvation daily, and these are the sins I have bumped into; ones that are not of God. I have bumped into sin in my life as a pastor and as a believer filled with the Holy Ghost. I bump into stuff in me that is straight out of hell. It ought not to be. So let us deal with it. Hallelujah.

Going back to Hebrews 4:13, it says, "Neither is there any creature that is not manifest in his sight: but all things are naked and opened unto the eyes of him with whom we have to do."

Neither is there any creature that is not manifest in his sight: but all things are naked and opened unto the eyes of him with whom we have to do. Hebrews 4:13 KJV

ALL THINGS ARE VISIBLE

Now we have light meeting darkness. So what is the creature? Is that a human being running around? Someone may say, "Well, that is just the devil." No, but he has a kingdom. Remember the old recruitment posters from World War II, with Uncle Sam on them? They said: "I need you." Well, Uncle Satan says, "I need you." Every principality from Satan's kingdom says, "I need you because without you I do not have a reason for existence. I cannot manifest myself by my fallen nature. I am stuck in this dry place of torment. I have every urge for evil. I have every urge because that is my nature, and no way to manifest it. I will find me a human."

As a result, our land and our world is filled with tragedy. The good news is that God has not given us a spirit of fear but of power, love, and a sound mind.

> *For God hath not given us the spirit of fear; but of power, and of love, and of a sound mind. 2 Timothy 1:7 KJV*

My mind is becoming one with my spirit, and my spirit is becoming one with God so that the Scriptures may be fulfilled. "For as many as are led by the Spirit of God, they are the sons of God."

> *For as many as are led by the Spirit of God, they are the sons of God. Romans 8:14 KJV*

As we learn to follow Father God, there is no creature that is not made manifest before our eyes, but all things are visible and naked — not only in my own life but in others' too. That is why *discerning of spirits* is one of the nine gifts of the Holy Spirit. What good is it to discern spirits if we cannot deal with them? Someone may say, "Well, I am into discerning of spirits." Whoopie, congratulations! That is the equivalent of declaring, "I have 14 roaches on my floor." We may have 14 roaches, but what are we going to do with them if they are in our house? Romans 16:20 says, "And the God of peace shall bruise Satan under your feet shortly."

> *And the God of peace shall bruise Satan under your feet shortly. The grace of our Lord Jesus Christ be with you. Amen. Romans 16:20 KJV*

Get that roach under our feet. When we see it, we can say, "Bless God, I see you, you roach," and we can address the problem. Sometimes we may see parts of our nature and personality that reflect the nature of the devil. But how is the nature of the devil made manifest? Through the body of sin. Have we not heard the Scripture about the *body of sin*? We have heard about the Body of Christ, have we not? Do we remember reading about the body of sin in Scripture?

> *Knowing this, that our old man is crucified with him, that the body of sin might be destroyed, that henceforth we should not serve sin. Romans 6:6 KJV*

Is the Body of Christ just one member? No, it is many members. What is the body of sin? It is also comprised of many members. How does God operate on this planet? Through us. How does Satan operate on this planet? Through us. It is reality check time. A true test of spirituality is found in Hebrews 5:14, which says that strong meat belongs to them, "who by reason of use have their senses exercised to discern both good and evil."

> *But strong meat belongeth to them that are of full age, even those who by reason of use have their senses exercised to discern both good and evil. Hebrews 5:14 KJV*

Someone may say they are afraid of evil. Shame on them. They may also say, "Well, I do not want to think about evil." Shame on them. Do we know what the Word says about our God? It says that light and darkness are the same to him.

> *Yea, the darkness hideth not from thee; but the night shineth as the day: the darkness and the light are both alike to thee. Psalm 139:12 KJV*

What does it mean that light and darkness are the same to Him? It means that our God is not intimidated by darkness. In fact, David said even if he made his bed in hell, God was there.

> *If I ascend up into heaven, thou art there: if I make my bed in hell, behold, thou art there. Psalm 139:8 KJV*

Did Jesus go to hell? He did not stay there, but He preached to the disobedient spirits from the days of Noah.

> [18] *For Christ also hath once suffered for sins, the just for the unjust, that he might bring us to God, being put to death in the flesh, but quickened by the Spirit:* [19]*By which also he went and preached unto the spirits in prison;* [20]*Which sometime were disobedient, when once the longsuffering of God waited in the days of Noah, while the ark was a preparing, wherein few, that is, eight souls were saved by water. 1 Peter 3:18-20 KJV*

He also spoiled principalities and powers. Of course, we will not go to hell to preach to disobedient spirits. But we need to confront "hell" in our own lives. During certain seasons, it is time for us to take a walk into the hell of our lives and stop pretending it is not there. We need to take up our armor. Let us take the helmet of salvation, our loins gird about with truth, with the breastplate of righteousness, shield of faith, and the sword of the spirit.

What is the sword of the spirit? It is the Word of God. Remember how Jesus defeated Satan? By saying, "For it is written," and quoting back Scriptures. The churches today are quoting "For it is written," but they have not been obedient to the Word they are trying to implement. They are unsanctified saints trying to bring forth the fruit of sanctification, and we cannot have the fruit without repentance. Remember what 2 Corinthians 10:6 says? "Having in a readiness to revenge all disobedience, when your obedience is fulfilled."

And having in a readiness to revenge all disobedience, when your obedience is fulfilled. 2 Corinthians 10:6 KJV

CORRECT SPIRITUAL WARFARE

We have no more power over the enemy in and of ourselves. Our power over the enemy is no greater than our obedience to the Word of God. It is He who fights on our behalf when we follow Him. And the churches today are trying to do so many spiritual warfare programs, but they, in their own lives, are not obedient to God's Word. How do I know that? Because in Deuteronomy 28 under curses, there is a long list of diseases. All the diseases listed there are because of separation from God and His Word. As people refuse to follow His instruction and follow sin instead, they have the consequences manifested in their bodies. So if I find a saint with a disease, I know they are separated from God and His Word. Even if they are trying to do spiritual warfare, they will not have the power because God is not going to honor just the Word without obedience. He will honor our obedience to the Word, in that, He honors us and it at the same time. We not only pray in His name, but we must also apply His Word to our lives.

*I will worship toward thy holy temple,
and praise thy name for thy
lovingkindness and for thy truth: for
thou hast magnified thy word above all
thy name. Psalm 138:2 KJV*

I have book after book on my shelves from the
New Age and false religions and cults of all kinds,
and every one quotes Scripture at some level. Does it
bother us if we run into an evil book that quotes
Scripture? It probably offends us. It challenges us and
makes us "nervous and jerky". But do not be nervous
and jerky because Satan quoted the Word to Eve, and
he quoted it to Jesus. And if he quoted it to Eve
wrong and he quoted it to Jesus wrong, what do we
think he does to us? Do we believe we are immune to
the evil one coming with his kingdom and lying to
us? Not at all.

Going back to Mark 7, beginning in verse 20, it
says, "And he said, That which cometh out of the
man, that defileth the man. For from within, out of the
heart of men, proceed evil thoughts."

*²⁰And he said, That which cometh out of
the man, that defileth the man. ²¹For
from within, out of the heart of men,
proceed evil thoughts, adulteries,
fornications, murders, ²²Thefts,
covetousness, wickedness, deceit,
lasciviousness, an evil eye, blasphemy,
pride, foolishness: ²³All these evil things
come from within, and defile the man.
Mark 7:20-23 KJV*

Where does evil proceed from? The heart of man. It does not say soul, does it? Evil thoughts do not have their beginning "upstairs" in our minds. They have their beginning in the very depths of our human spirits. Where do the evil spirits that are in place in our lives come from? "For from within, out of the heart of men, proceed evil thoughts, adulteries, fornications, murders, Thefts, covetousness, wickedness, deceit, lasciviousness, an evil eye, blasphemy, pride, foolishness: All these evil things come from within and defile the man."

Chapter 7: How to Recover Ourselves

BE CONFORMED TO HIS IMAGE

So, that leaves us with the question of how we recover ourselves out of these snares. Hebrews 12:15 says, "Looking diligently lest any man fail of the grace of God; lest any root of bitterness springing up trouble you, and thereby many others be defiled."

Looking diligently lest any man fail of the grace of God; lest any root of bitterness springing up trouble you, and thereby many be defiled; Hebrews 12:15 KJV

Where does the root of bitterness settle into? Right into our human spirit. Someone may object that it is an evil spirit. Let us mark this down—I do not want to make Satan's kingdom and its operation vague. I want to carefully mark down a specific aspect of God's Kingdom versus Satan's. Every aberration of God's nature, known as sin, is supported by a specific evil spirit that manifests its nature. Their purpose in manifesting in our lives is so that the body of sin may be manifested in the earth through humans. However, God has called us out of that darkness into His marvelous light. He has called us out of death into life so that we could be raised up to the praise of His glory, that we would establish His righteousness on the earth. It comes out of our willing obedience to choose to follow Him.

But ye are a chosen generation, a royal priesthood, an holy nation, a peculiar people; that ye should shew forth the praises of him who hath called you out of darkness into his marvellous light; 1 Peter 2:9 KJV

In other words, Father God wants us to follow Him out of our own heart's desire. Not because we are afraid that He will strike us down or a curse will come into our lives, but because we want to obey Him. This is about making a quality decision for our own lives, not to follow Satan's kingdom. We are a Holy Ghost "love bug" without any guile in our hearts. I mean that we love to the degree that we pay no attention to wrongs done unto us. We are filled with faith and therefore have no bitterness, envy and jealousy, fear, self-hatred, rejection, guilt, condemnation, adultery, or lust. We are a reflection of Father God Himself walking on the earth.

Do we have a way to go? Do we feel condemned in it? Satan is trying to make us one with sin and our failings if we do. But if my words bring conviction as a breath of life, we can separate ourselves from those sins and look at ourselves according to the truth. As we grow in our understanding of being a new creature, we must understand that we are on a journey. Growing into a new creature requires remembering that we have yet to arrive at the stature of measure of what that represents. Have we arrived yet?

I had somebody a few years ago inform me that they were sinless and had no sin. I thought to myself, "Boy, have we got a problem here." We confronted that individual with at least nine or ten evil spirits that we could observe in them. Their response, when confronted, they said: "No, I am born again. I am a new creature. I do not have any evil in me whatsoever." Well, what do we do with that? We cannot help anyone unwilling to consider whether they have sin or not. The only way this journey works is if we walk in the light, as He is in the light, we have fellowship one with another, and the blood of Jesus cleanses us from all unrighteousness.

> *But if we walk in the light, as he is in the light, we have fellowship one with another, and the blood of Jesus Christ his Son cleanseth us from all sin. 1 John 1:7 KJV*

In the world we live in today, two Scriptural laws compete for our attention. One Kingdom operates according to the Word of God, but the other openly defies it. Satan's kingdom rules by lawlessness. Paul, when writing to the church at Rome, stated that we become slaves to the ones we obey — either God or Satan.

> *[22]For I delight in the law of God after the inward man: [23]But I see another law in my members, warring against the law*

*of my mind, and bringing me into
captivity to the law of sin which is in
my members. [24]O wretched man that I
am! who shall deliver me from the body
of this death? [25]I thank God through
Jesus Christ our Lord. So then with the
mind I myself serve the law of God; but
with the flesh the law of sin. Romans
7:22-25 KJV*

As we choose to serve Father God, we are
being conformed unto the image of our Lord, Jesus
Christ.

*[10]That I may know him, and the power
of his resurrection, and the fellowship of
his sufferings, being made conformable
unto his death; [11]If by any means I
might attain unto the resurrection of the
dead. Philippians 3:10-11 KJV*

WE ARE NOT A FINISHED PRODUCT

Our conversation has centered on who we are
after conversion and being formed into sons and
daughters of God. Who were we before conversion?
Our identity may not have changed much after we
were born again. We may be struggling with some of
the same problems that we struggled with before
conversion. Now, this may grate against our flesh a
little bit; however, it is important to challenge what
we believe about ourselves and those around us.
Humanity today is a mixture of the nature of God and

the nature of the devil—including the Christian Church, whether we choose to face that truth or not. If that were not the case, then we would not need sanctification. If we were not facing problems in our lives, we would not need sanctification. So, what are we being sanctified from? What did Paul mean in 2 Corinthians 7:1? It begins, "Having therefore these promises, dearly beloved."

> *Having therefore these promises, dearly beloved, let us cleanse ourselves from all filthiness of the flesh and spirit, perfecting holiness in the fear of God. 2 Corinthians 7:1 KJV*

What are *these promises*? The promises of freedom in Christ. If freedom in Christ was already a finished product for us at the cross, why do we need promises? Indeed what Christ did at the cross was a finished work for all of mankind. When Jesus died for the sins of the world, it was a finished work. However, is everyone saved? No. Then how could Jesus say it was finished? He finished it and established it, but what is missing? The appropriation of many humans in the present. Much of the modern Church is teaching that everything was finished; therefore, we do not need to appropriate, by repentance, what was finished at the cross. As a result, we are messed up because of those teachings. Many people are living in denial because they have the consequences of sin in their lives through insanity and disease, and they ignore the root of the problem—sin.

Now, we are caught in a paradox of theology. What is the paradox of theology? The Bible promises that we are free in Christ, but our lives do not reflect that freedom. As a result, we struggle with guilt and condemnation. The devil hits us with memories in our minds as sort-of "flashcards" of our present and past. We are tormented because, on one hand, we are told it was a finished work. And at the same time, we are not walking in that finished product. Then if we dare question our leadership about this subject, they simply tell us, "Have more faith." However, why would we need faith for something that is already finished? Scriptures state, "Faith is the substance of things hoped for, the evidence of things not seen."

Now faith is the substance of things hoped for, the evidence of things not seen. Hebrews 11:1 KJV

Faith projects into the future a currently incomplete work. So why would we need faith for something that is already finished and complete? We do not need faith for something that is already finished. That is a ridiculous position. It is absurd and intellectually makes no sense. We do not need faith for something that is finished. However, this is where appropriation is important for our faith. We can appropriate the finished work at the cross by faith as a provision for our lives.

KEEP HIS COMMANDMENTS

But how do we appropriate the Word of God? By obedience. There is that terrible word: obedience. If there is any anti-Christ spirit within any person, they will be riled up at the word *obedience*. And if we are not careful, we will be accused of legalism if we mention the word. Jesus said if we loved Him, we would keep His commandments.

> *If ye love me, keep my commandments.*
> *John 14:15 KJV*

If obedience equates to legalism, then Jesus would be the greatest legalist of all. However, Jesus does not demand obedience by force. Does He come and hit us over the head with that commandment? Did Jesus force us to be born again? Did the Father force us to become a son or daughter of God? Does the Father, the Lord Jesus, and the Holy Spirit force us to do anything? I cannot make someone do anything against their will. If I tried to force someone to obey the Word of God, I would have a revolt on my hands. I would have anarchy.

God has created us with free will. However, even though Jesus defeated the devil at the cross as a finished work, it does not mean we have done the same. If the Lord had not died for our sins, there would be no provision for the forgiveness of sin. Without the shedding of blood, there is no remission of sins. We can probably quote that Scripture from memory.

*And almost all things are by the law
purged with blood; and without
shedding of blood is no remission.
Hebrews 9:22 KJV*

*²⁷And he took the cup, and gave thanks,
and gave it to them, saying, Drink ye all
of it; ²⁸For this is my blood of the new
testament, which is shed for many for
the remission of sins. Matthew 26:27-28
KJV*

If Jesus had not died as a sacrificial Lamb at the
cross, we would still be dead in our trespasses and
sins. We cannot earn our way out of that conclusion
by religious works. I do not care how many churches
a person goes to, how many church services they go
to, how many religions they create; they would still
be separated from God without Jesus' shed blood.
That is how God ordained it, whether we like it or
not. However, just because Jesus shed His blood at
the cross, not all humans have appropriated it, have
they? Regardless of their decision not to repent and
believe, is it still a finished product? Was it finished
from the foundation of the world? Was it finished at
the cross? If it is a finished work, what do we have to
do? Appropriate it.

WHY ARE WE SICK?

Now, how does this subject relate to healing?
Remember that by His stripes, we are healed.

But he was wounded for our transgressions, he was bruised for our iniquities: the chastisement of our peace was upon him; and with his stripes we are healed. Isaiah 53:5 KJV

Who his own self bare our sins in his own body on the tree, that we, being dead to sins, should live unto righteousness: by whose stripes ye were healed. 1 Peter 2:24 KJV

Some believers take that statement and say, "Well, all healing was provided for 2,000 years ago, and therefore, I am no longer sick." At the same time, they are still sick. If healing is a finished product, why are we sick? It would seem that the minute we became born again, every demon in hell would flee, but they did not. Not only did they not flee, but they were stirred up even more after we became believers. I have heard more people tell me, "I did not have all these problems until I was born again." That is not a true statement. The reality is that we were in total darkness, and we did not know we were dying. After being born again, we know we are dying and are tormented by it.

I have heard more people say, "Well, I do not know if I should serve the Lord. I did not have these problems before I came to God." And I look at them and say, "Do you know what? As a Christian, the sin manifesting in you would have been destroyed your life had you not been saved. The evil spirits were already there. They did not come into you when you became born again. And the best thing that can happen to you, you may not like what I will say next, is the stuff starting to stir up. However, what happens to you when it gets stirred up is that you are not able to separate yourself from it, and you sink down under it. And the devil intends that you do so. His first point of attack is that he wants to ensure that you do not realize that it was finished at the cross. Number two, he wants to ensure that you do not separate yourself from his nature in your life."

Satan wants to be the head of the Church. Forget about just being the god of this world; he wants to be the head of the Church. He wants to be the head of everything that represents God. I am not moved by people and their religious clichés because Satan is a great cliché. When Jesus was tempted in Luke 4, Satan quoted Scripture from Deuteronomy and Psalms. He perverted it when he quoted and took it out of context. When Eve was tempted, Satan came and quoted the Word of God to Eve—but he changed it.

Back in the days of Adam and Eve, the Bible involved one Scripture. The Bible was one verse long: Do not eat of the fruit of the tree of the knowledge of good and evil. Period. That was it. Would we like to have a Bible that long? In the Garden of Eden, a Bible study was short. "Thou shall not eat of the fruit of the knowledge of good and evil." And that would be our Bible study every single day. Sadly, they did not follow it. And all it took was for Satan, through the medium of a serpent, to question that one Scripture—

and Eve chose to disobey God. Not only did Satan change the Word, but he also added to and questioned Scripture in order to deceive her.

So, now we must address how appropriation functions in our lives. Someone may say, "Okay, I am going to appropriate salvation, and I am going to appropriate healing." However, if we appropriate healing *philosophically* and are not healed immediately, we may believe we have a problem. What do we do then? Maybe we create a new doctrine that God does not heal today. The logic behind this decision might be: "If He healed today, He would have healed me." However, appropriation is not an instantaneous change; it is a lifetime journey. Our lives and entire generation is a continual transformation of all three dimensions of our existence. Someone may ask me to prove it to them. Oh, that is easy. First Thessalonians 5:23 begins by saying that the God of peace will sanctify us. Sanctification is God's car wash. God is the potter, and we are the clay. I am the gold, and He is the fire. And what comes to the surface when they put the gold in the fire, and it liquefies? The dross or the impurity.

LED BY THE SPIRIT

We are to be refined as fine gold. This church ministry stands for refining people as fine gold instead of hyping them up on promises so they feel like they have been given a parachute to jump off the church steeple and say they are "flying in the Spirit".

We do not begin in the Spirit and end in the flesh. We begin in the Spirit and we stay in the Spirit. The Bible does not say, "For as many as are led by the flesh are the sons of God." No, it says: "For as many as are led by the Spirit of God, they are the sons of God."

For as many as are led by the Spirit of God, they are the sons of God. Romans 8:14 KJV

I have a couple of stories that serve as examples of how to operate as sons and daughters of God in normal, day-to-day life. We had to go to pick up a twenty-one-foot travel trailer at 7:00 at night. We drove up to Fayetteville, Georgia. We were driving an old Ford pickup truck, barreling down the highway. We arrived at the house, and there was a big, giant hitch to pull the trailer. The problem was that it took a 2 5/16th-inch ball and we had a 2-inch ball on the pickup. Some men came over to help us and said we could not attach this to the back of our truck.

We left the trailer and rushed to find an auto discount store to buy another ball for the rear bumper. We found an auto parts store with a 2 5/16th-inch ball. The lady behind the counter loaned us a wrench. As we went to take the old one off, we found the new one would not fit. The hole in the steel bumper was too small. The one that needed to go in had a 1-inch thread, and the hole was only ¾-inch, and it was a solid steel bumper — there was no way to force the bolt into the hole.

It was 7:15 at night or later. So, I said, "Well, we need to drive down the road. We have to find a way to cut this hole larger." We began driving down the road and we came up to a four-way turn. We were considering where we should go next without a specific direction. Shall we go left? I put it in the left lane to turn. Then I stopped and said, "I do not want to go this way. I think we should go this other way. What we need are some construction workers who just got off work. They must have a cutting torch in the back of their truck, sitting alongside the road."

We drove along looking for someone. I had faith that Father God would provide for us. We were about a mile down the road and saw all these construction trucks sitting on the side of the road. I saw a compressor and thought maybe it was a cutting torch. That instant, I saw an acetylene tank sitting on this other truck. So we pulled in there. We wandered up to the workers, and they looked at us like, "Who are you?" And I said, "Guys, we need some help. We need somebody to cut a hole in the back of this bumper to attach this metal ball. Can you do that?" They looked at each other, and one guy said, "I reckon we could."

Two minutes later, the job was done. From the time we had left the other house to go look for a ball, it was thirty minutes. In that time, we took the old ball off and saw it was too small, went back into the store, returned the new ball along with the wrench, drove down the road and had the hole cut into the solid steel bumper, drove back to the store to buy the new ball and borrowed their wrench again, and finally arrived back at the house. We had a deadline because we had to be back by dark, and we pulled onto the property just in time. Just because we follow God does not mean we will not face hurdles and challenges. The difference is in what we do with those obstacles. Father God provided a means to complete a task that may have seemed unsurmountable at the time. And so, all things work together for good to them who love the Lord and are called according to His purposes.

> *And we know that all things work together for good to them that love God, to them who are the called according to his purpose. Romans 8:28 KJV*

That was an event I will never forget. It was incredible. It was a practical example of being led by the Spirit of God. For context, Fayetteville was a smaller town, and at 7:30 at night we were looking for somebody who could cut a hole in solid steel. All the shops were closed. All the garages were closed. Everyone who could help with our task was closed, and exactly what we were looking for came to my mind. We needed some guys hanging out with a cutting torch, and I said, "Let us just keep driving; we will find them." That is an excellent testimony to Father God's faithfulness.

MIRACULOUS PROVISION

I have experienced the miraculous in my life. I remember events that happened as I was learning to know and trust God. They were incredible and miraculous, yet they would happen in normal, everyday events. May I share another testimony? For years, I ran an industrial sharpening service specializing in all kinds of carbide, cutting, and saw blades. I worked with anything that needed to be sharpened. I did that for 13 years, and I owned the business. I had just come to the Lord. Up until that time, we were working seven days a week. We worked from 7:00 in the morning to around 10:00 at night. I was doing well financially with a big, fancy home.

The first week I came to the Lord, I faced a challenge because my church had services on Thursday nights. Friday was our big delivery day in construction because it was the day everyone was paid. The contractors received their money, and Friday, we loaded up on deliveries because that was when we would also be paid. The rest of the week, there was no cash to be made. I had certain charge accounts with us, but many paid with cash or wrote checks. If I did not get to them within that one or two hours of receiving their money, I had to wait a week to obtain payment. At the same time, I had to make payroll and expenses that required payment, and I had to get these done by Thursday night. However, now, I also had church services on Thursday nights.

When I came to God, I really committed to

of me. It was not as if I just turning a page; I was not the same man anymore. I did not even think the same way anymore. It was scary because we are conditioned in ways of thinking and pressure to make a living and take care of business. That week was a busy week in our shop, and we had three large orders of blades to be sharpened. The blades for those three orders would have taken at least an hour and a half each if we just had one man assigned to production. It would have taken three men an hour and a half to two hours to finish these three orders, which were scheduled to be delivered on the next day — Friday. It also represented several hundred dollars of income we needed for payroll.

We worked right up until 5:00, and I was looking at these stacks of blades, thinking, "Oh, my goodness. We need the money. We could stay here until about 7:30 or 8:00 and finish it off, but we would miss church." At the same time, I had decided that when church was open, I would be there because I wanted to be fed. I was hungry to learn the Word of God and His ways. When I was born again, years of frustration were peeling off of me. I looked at the crew, and I said, "Nope, we are not finishing; we are going to church. This is my decision. I am going to shut down this operation, go home, get myself cleaned up, get dinner, and we are going to church. We will just make a delivery on Monday or Tuesday or whenever we are finished. I will take the consequences." I closed the operation and went to church. As a reminder, this is a true story. I am not exaggerating it. We returned the following day and opened up at 7:00 in the morning, and all of those blades were completely done. They were sharpened and sitting there ready for delivery, and not one member of my crew did it. I am telling the truth.

All I can say is that angels know how to sharpen saw blades. I will look for that crew of angels one day and say, "Boys, how did you do that?" There were three huge stacks of blades that were totally dirty — when blades are dirty, they are very dirty. When we walked in, they were clean and sharp. Tickets in order, and ready for delivery. Not one person in my staff did them. That got my attention.

Here is another story to strengthen our faith. My uncles and people in my family tree were pastors and missionaries. Two of my uncles were modern-day apostles in Africa, each establishing over 1,000 African churches. As a kid, I remember one of my uncles coming back on furlough and telling us an incredible story. They were in the bush driving from one little place to another and were scheduled to minister to a bush tribe. This event took place back in the 1950's, and there were no roads at that time; there were just ruts. They had had some rain that day. The rain came and went, and they were in the middle of nowhere.

They were scheduled to meet that very day, and they were out in the bush bogged down in a mud hole in the ruts and could not get out. In trying to get out, they used all their gas and were stranded in the middle of nowhere. Their wheels were stuck up to the axle in mud, and they were stranded without gas.

They prayed and asked God to get them to the meeting so they could bring the Gospel to this tribe. When they finished the prayer, as they were sitting in the vehicle, it started moving, and the motor was not running. The vehicle came out of the mud, and they steered it all the way to the village without the motor running over many miles. This is a story that I grew up with as a child. I never forgot that testimony of how God could sovereignly do this.

SIMPLICITY OF FAITH

As I have been sharing these examples of faith, it is important to remember the simplicity of it. We often need to return to a childlike faith when we pray and make requests to Father God. Sometimes our minds get in the middle of our faith and overcomplicate our journey. I believe God loves it if we become childlike in our faith. We have become so sophisticated with our models of spiritual warfare that we forget to simply ask for what we need. My children do not go through one hour of spiritual warfare to get a quarter or two from me. They do not fast and pray for three days. They just come and ask me for a quarter.

Years ago, one of my younger daughters had trouble taking her naps. I had to leave, and when I returned, I asked, "Did you take your nap without causing trouble and discontent for a few hours?" She had been obedient without causing trouble going down for her nap. I was so proud of her that I reached into my pocket and dug out two quarters, and said,

"Here, Baby, here are a couple of quarters." She loved quarters because the mechanical horses that could be ridden at Walmart required quarters. She would say she wanted "big money", as in quarters, which are larger coins. She did not want nickels, dimes, or pennies. She only wanted "big money," so I gave her two quarters for two rides at Walmart. When I gave it to her, she said, "Me? Daddy, are the quarters for me because I was obedient?" At first, I said, "Well, yes, in a way, but just because I love you, okay?" However, I changed my position slightly because I did not want to tie my gift to her performance. I said, "No, I gave you the 'big money' just because I love you. But I really do appreciate that you obey me." She smiled. About 15 or 20 minutes later, she approached me and asked, "Dad, if I am obedient to you in more ways, can I have more quarters?" I looked at her and said, "I will give you quarters anyway, Baby, so do not worry about it. But, I certainly appreciate your obedience." I wanted to model to her what I have observed about Father God. We do not obey to get what we want from Him. However, if we appreciate Father God and love Him, we will obey Him because we want to follow Him.

I have a final example to amplify my main point. After I came to the Lord, I was still working in my saw business, and I had an old Ford Econoline that used a quart of oil every 50 miles. It would regularly leak out. I went to start it one day, and it had already used up around 10-12 quarts of oil. My problem was that I did not have enough cash to pay for more, with only two dollars left in my pocket. Oil was pouring out, and I found myself 90 miles from my office on empty without enough money to fill up.

I was supposed to meet with a customer, and it did not appear I would make it. This particular customer eventually was born again, but he was really nasty at that time. If I promised to meet him and did not keep my word to show up on time, he would not just cuss me out—he would *really* cuss me out. And then he would go to a competitor and torment me for a month or two and then come back and laugh at me. This guy was tough. As the saying goes, he would "eat nails for breakfast." I had a delivery scheduled by the end of the day because he needed it for the next day. I had his order on my van, I was almost 90 miles away, and it was late in the afternoon. I put my last two dollars of gas in the tank, knowing it would get me about 30 or 40 miles. I had to make a detour in about eight or ten miles to get to this job by 4:30 in the afternoon, and then I had another 35-mile drive back to my office. Seeing the challenge in front of me, I started to pray.

So here I was driving, and I started to pray earnestly, asking for help. I said, "God, I must get to this job site, and I am a man of integrity. I keep my word if I can, but this guy will not find it acceptable if I am late. So, God, here is my prayer, I want You to extend the gas in the tank as I drive." This vehicle also leaked oil, and I had just used the last of my money. Realizing this, I said, "God, keep this vehicle going and keep the valves lubricated somehow so my motor is not damaged. Please, take me to the job and my house because it will be late by that time. I will not go to the office. I just want to make it to the house. Please, take me home and let me go to the job site. And, Lord, I will just drive and forget about the gas issue." In my mind, the gas gauge was right in front of me, but I determined that I would not focus on the gas gauge and trust Father God instead. Even with two dollars of gas in the tank, it was still on empty. The vehicle's gauge was on the little black line near empty, and if I did not find a gas station in half of a mile, I would be walking because it would not go anywhere. It had left me stranded before, so I knew what could happen.

With that in mind, but determined to trust God, I started to drive. I drove 10 miles; then 15 miles; 20 miles; 30 miles; and 40 miles. When I came to where the interstate split with eight or nine miles to the job, I had a decision to make. At that point, one part of me said, "Go home." The other part said, "He is waiting for you." Then I remembered my prayer. I decided to go to the job site. I arrived at 4:30 and was able to give the guy his saw blades; he was happy, and I did not have to listen to his tirade. I returned to my van and started driving. Now, I had 35 more miles to go. I had already gone 55 miles, and I was still driving 35 more miles. Suddenly, I started to get excited because I knew there was no gas in that truck. It was impossible for it to have driven that far, and I had 35 miles to go, which was a long way. The more I drove, the more excited I became.

I kept driving, and by this time, if it had run out of gas, I would have still been thankful. I was a happy Henry. Faith had been quickened in me, and I drove; I kept driving and looking around. I pulled off the interstate and drove into town, watching my prayer come to pass as I drew closer to my home. It happened years ago, but it is still incredibly clear to me today. As I turned down the road to my house, I turned my wheels to go into my driveway. It stopped running, and I coasted right into the driveway as the engine died at my home, and there it sat. I sat there for a moment savoring this incredible journey, and everything I believed for had come to pass.

I do not drive around without enough gas trying to replicate that event because that would be tempting God — but I believe that He is not that far away from us. I suspect sometimes we become so set in our ways that we do not allow ourselves to become like children in our faith. I think we need to cultivate, not necessarily be naive, but we need to go back to those earlier days of our faith. I have seen God perform miracles for "baby" Christians that He never does anymore for mature Christians. In some ways, I would prefer to stay a "baby" Christian than a mature one because it is more fun. Do we remember those early days when we first came to the Lord? Do we remember many of the things we were believing for, and how a lot of them came to pass? Then the more mature we became, they did not happen anymore. Did we ever notice that? Why did they quit happening? Did God stop loving us? I think we became too sophisticated in our believing and faith, and the enemy came to program us with unbelief and doubt. Part of our identity requires a return to the simplicity of faith that began our journeys. Perhaps, Father God is waiting for us to trust Him rather than figure out everything for ourselves.

Chapter 8: Two Kingdoms

WE ARE NOT EVIL

It is disconcerting to many people when I start to discuss that they might have evil as part of their existence. Maybe the devil accuses us of evil, or we see it for ourselves. Or perhaps it is pointed out in ministry that we have aspects of our thinking and nature that reflect the devil instead of God. Does that bother us? If it does, there are only two options in front of us. We can either go into denial and condemnation or go into conviction by God. Condemnation makes us one with evil, but conviction comes to separate us from evil. The devil does not just want us to feel guilty about sin in our lives, but he wants us to believe it is an inseparable part of who we are on the inside. The devil does not want to give us up and let God transform us. Which part do we want? Condemnation makes us one with evil. But conviction separates us from evil because the Holy Spirit shows us sin and leads us to repent so we can be free from that evil spirit. We are not evil; evil has joined us in our lives.

Throughout this text, I have referred to "the devil" and our lives, but he does not take a personal interest in us specifically. Satan does not currently inhabit any person. He is also not omnipresent. On the other hand, the Holy Spirit inhabits every person who is born again. He is omnipresent because He is the third member of the eternal Godhead. Jesus does not indwell us and live in us personally. God, the Father, does not live in us personally. The Holy Spirit lives in us personally, bearing witness of the Godhead.

Father God and the Word are one in the eternal Godhead. When people say they have "Jesus in their hearts", does that mean He lives in them personally? No, that would be impossible. Because not only is Jesus a Spirit since He is a member of the Godhead as God the Word, but since He became a human, He also has a personal human spirit. I know what I am writing may be challenging, but Jesus is not only a member of the eternal Godhead indivisible with God, but He also has a personal human spirit. He is all God and all man. God the Father is not a human. The Holy Spirit is not a human. But who exists as all God and all man today? The Son of God, Christ Jesus.

KINGS AND PRIESTS

He is Jesus, the Christ, but He is still God the Word. Not only is He part of the eternal Godhead, but He also has a personal spirit. When people are raised from the dead, do they exist as a personal spirit? In other words, will our human spirit still exist when we are raised from the dead? We will still be ourselves. Is Jesus still Jesus? Zechariah 13 shows Jesus during His millennial reign sitting in Jerusalem. They will see the scars that are still in His hands, and they will ask where He got those scars.

And one shall say unto him, What are
these wounds in thine hands? Then he
shall answer, Those with which I was
wounded in the house of my friends.
Zechariah 13:6 KJV

This message is prophetic and future tense.
This event has yet to happen because Jesus is not
currently ruling out of Jerusalem. When He returns to
the planet on the Day of the Lord, sets up His
Millennial Kingdom, and reigns in Jerusalem with the
saints, the nations will come and submit to Him. They
will come and submit to Him worldwide, and Kings
and Priests will administer that Kingdom. Those
Kings and Priests are us, along with all the Old and
New Testament saints. This is where we are headed.
That is our destiny as born-again believers—Kings
and Priests unto our God.

> *⁵And from Jesus Christ, who is the*
> *faithful witness, and the first begotten*
> *of the dead, and the prince of the kings*
> *of the earth. Unto him that loved us,*
> *and washed us from our sins in his own*
> *blood, ⁶And hath made us kings and*
> *priests unto God and his Father; to him*
> *be glory and dominion for ever and ever.*
> *Amen. Revelation 1:5-6 KJV*

Yet, in those days, Jesus will still have the scars
in His hands. And they will say, "Sir, where did You
get these scars and wounds?" And He will say,
"These are the wounds I received in the house of my
friends." Have we been in some battles with our

friends and family? Do we feel as if they have targeted us? Jesus has been there. He came to His own, and His own received Him not. His own murdered Him to fulfill the will of God.

> *¹⁰He was in the world, and the world was made by him, and the world knew him not. ¹¹He came unto his own, and his own received him not. John 1:10-11 KJV*

In His hands—in His glorified body—the scars are still there. How do I know that? Because Zechariah 13 is prophetic; it has not yet happened. So it is a future-tense event, and the question that is asked and answered will surely occur in that day. The question will be asked by someone, and His reply to them will be exactly as prophesied. It will be word for word. And there He will show His scars.

This is not my main point, but showing a glimpse of our eternal future is important. In this present time, we do not see what will be in the Millennial Reign, but God is with us right now. The Holy Spirit inhabits us. He is with every believer because God is omnipresent, or everywhere, at once. God, the Holy Spirit, is omnipresent. Is Satan omnipresent? Are evil spirits omnipresent? No. We talk about Satan, but he is not omnipresent. However, he administers a kingdom of beings. They are specifically detailed in Ephesians 6. They are principalities and powers, the rulers of the darkness of this world, and spiritual wickedness in high places.

For we wrestle not against flesh and blood, but against principalities, against powers, against the rulers of the darkness of this world, against spiritual wickedness in high places. Ephesians 6:12 KJV

He administers a kingdom of invisible, disembodied beings that want to inhabit humans. They want to enslave us to follow their desires. Paul was writing to the church at Rome when he stated that we become slaves to whomever we obey. We become slaves to God, which leads to conformity to Christ's character, righteousness, and holiness. Or we become slaves to rebellion, which leads to conformity to the image of Satan, death, and destruction. A repentant heart always opens the doorway for revelation from God. Those who repented under the ministry of John the Baptist recognized and welcomed Christ. The Pharisees and Sadducees, who were full of pride, self-righteousness, and importance, did not perceive the time of their visitation but rejected Jesus Christ, the Son of God. They did not realize the fulfillment of Scripture because they were blinded by sin.

ESTABLISHED BY FAITH

Now, I intend to challenge some notions of Scripture by moving over to Romans 6. It is important to bring Romans 6 into context by reading verses 1-6:

¹What shall we say then? Shall we continue in sin, that grace may abound? ²God forbid. How shall we, that are dead to sin, live any longer therein? ³Know ye not, that so many of us as were baptized into Jesus Christ were baptized into his death? ⁴Therefore we are buried with him by baptism into death: that like as Christ was raised up from the dead by the glory of the Father, even so we also should walk in newness of life. ⁵For if we have been planted together in the likeness of his death, we shall be also in the likeness of his resurrection: ⁶Knowing this, that our old man is crucified with him, that the body of sin might be destroyed, that henceforth we should not serve sin.
Romans 6:1-6 KJV

As it moves into verse 6, it says, "Knowing this, that our old man is crucified with him, that the body of sin might be destroyed, that henceforth we should not serve sin." The key parts I want to draw out of verse 6 are "sin might be destroyed" and "we should not serve sin". These statements are present progressive. They are not statements of completed, past-tense events. Many people take these verses and make them a completed statement and a finished work, and that is where they make a mistake. The body of sin SHOULD be destroyed and we SHOULD not serve sin. However, in everyday life, is it possible we do not obey the Word of God and enter into sin?

To remove the present progressive nature of this Scripture would eliminate the work of sanctification. We would not need to be sanctified at all, and that would violate 1 Thessalonians 5:23 because it indicates the need to be sanctified *wholly* or fully. That is a journey of growth, NOT a completed work.

And the very God of peace sanctify you wholly; and I pray God your whole spirit and soul and body be preserved blameless unto the coming of our Lord Jesus Christ. 1 Thessalonians 5:23 KJV

If we embrace the present progressive growth of sanctification, we have a place to address spiritual warfare as we face challenges in our lives. Progressive growth results in the transformation of our inner man. It requires faith to continue to be conformed into the likeness of God. It requires faith to trust Father God to continue to remove sin from our lives. And it goes further than that. We are establishing the Kingdom of God in the midst of evil. It would be much easier if we could remove Satan and evil entirely from our lives and never be tempted by sin ever again. It would be much easier to establish the Kingdom of God without evil. However, as Satan continues to establish his kingdom in the midst of men, God is also establishing His Kingdom in the midst of men.

Both kingdoms are established by faith. Men serve Satan by faith, and men serve God by faith.

When men believe the lies of Satan's kingdom, they establish his ways on the earth. As we believe the truth of the Word of God according to Scripture, we establish God's Kingdom on earth. When we look around, it may appear Satan is winning in taking over the planet. However, God's great coup is taking normal humans like us, who have every reason to sin, to establish His Kingdom amid a kingdom of Satan and in spite of it. Amazingly, we defeat these invisible enemies through our obedience. If this war were fleshly and physical, we would have a fistfight with the enemy. However, the weapons of our warfare are not carnal. Our weapons of warfare are not carnal, but mighty to the pulling down of strongholds.

(For the weapons of our warfare are not carnal, but mighty through God to the pulling down of strong holds;) 2 Corinthians 10:4 KJV

WHO IS OUR MASTER?

Returning to Romans 6:6:

Knowing this, that our old man is crucified with him, that the body of sin might be destroyed, that henceforth we should not serve sin. Romans 6:6 KJV

What needs to be destroyed? The body of sin. Moving on to the next verses:

⁹Knowing that Christ being raised from the dead dieth no more; death hath no more dominion over him. ¹⁰For in that he died, he died unto sin once: but in that he liveth, he liveth unto God. ¹¹Likewise reckon ye also yourselves to be dead indeed unto sin, but alive unto God through Jesus Christ our Lord. ¹²Let not sin therefore reign in your mortal body, that ye should obey it in the lusts thereof. Romans 6:9-12 KJV

In verse 12, is Paul writing that sin does not exist in our mortal bodies, or is he indicating it *does* exist in our mortal bodies? He is indicating it *does* exist in our mortal bodies. This Scripture addresses present progressive. Paul is directing his comments to Christians, not referring to the unsaved. By saying, "Let not sin therefore reign in your mortal body," he indicates they have the option to follow God instead of sin. Additionally, he warns them not to let it reign in their bodies, which indicates that sin is already inside them.

So what are we to do with sin? Crucify it and put it to death. Get rid of it and be purified in our spirit, soul, and body that we should not obey it. Look at verse 13-14: "Neither yield ye your members as instruments of unrighteousness unto sin: but yield yourselves unto God, as those that are alive from the dead, and your members as instruments of righteousness unto God. For sin shall not have dominion over you."

[13]Neither yield ye your members as instruments of unrighteousness unto sin: but yield yourselves unto God, as those that are alive from the dead, and your members as instruments of righteousness unto God. [14]For sin shall not have dominion over you: for ye are not under the law, but under grace.
Romans 6:13-14 KJV

Does it say that sin will not try to have dominion over us? No, it does not. Does it say we will not be tempted? No. Does it say that we do not need to be sanctified? No, it only instructs us not to let sin be our master. Do not let Satan and his kingdom be master. Do not let fear be master. Do not let jealousy be master. Do not let an Unloving spirit be master. Do not let self-rejection and self-hatred be master. Do not let bitterness be master. Do not let anger be master. Do not let rage be master. Do not let violence be master. Do not let all these evil spirits from Satan's kingdom be master. We have the decision either to listen to Satan's kingdom or resist it.

According to verse 14, we have the ability to defeat sin. Before God was in our lives, we were dead in our tracks. However, remember that we are not automatically free. We must choose not to listen to Satan's kingdom and its thoughts. Verse 15 goes on to say, "What then? shall we sin, because we are not under the law, but under grace? God forbid."

What then? shall we sin, because we are
not under the law, but under grace? God
forbid. Romans 6:15 KJV

Moving on to verse 16, read carefully because this is where I am going in this conversation. "Know ye not, that to whom ye yield yourself servants to obey, his servants ye are to whom ye obey; whether of sin unto death, or of obedience unto righteousness?"

Know ye not, that to whom ye yield
yourselves servants to obey, his
servants ye are to whom ye obey;
whether of sin unto death, or of
obedience unto righteousness? Romans
6:16 KJV

If we obey the law of sin as Christians, it has become our master. We may declare "Jesus is Lord", but in the areas of our lives where we are bound in sin, He is not Lord. I know many Christians with spiritual problems—rage, anger, hatred, bitterness, and suspicion. In those areas, they are ruled by the devil.

Many people struggle over the subject of demon possession. Many people take the stance that a devil cannot possess a Christian. I agree with them. If an evil spirit or devil can possess a Christian, it indicates possession or total ownership. However, what people have done with this position is take it to another extreme. They have moved into another fallacy in their thought processes by reasoning that because an evil spirit cannot possess us, we cannot have an evil spirit in our lives. They have eliminated the kingdom of evil spirits and principalities, and now our enemy is only the devil himself—Satan.

Satan is not alone. He has an invisible kingdom described in Ephesians 6. This kingdom is very active in the world and answers to his authority. They desire to bring us under their submission to become our masters so that we become their slaves. If Christians cannot stop in anger, they are possessed by a spirit of anger, and to this degree, they have become its slave, and it has become their master. Why? Because a Christian has decided to follow after sin. God will not force us to come out of agreement with sin if we choose to participate with its thoughts. However, if a Christian is bound by a spirit of lust they cannot seem to get rid of, they are not immediately doomed to hell. They are bound in that area of their lives, but they are still born again. Jesus still loves them.

SIN IS A BEING

My point is not to focus on whether Christians can or cannot lose their salvation but to focus on that area of their lives where Jesus is not Lord. Satan, operating through his kingdom of evil spirits, is the lord over them. Lust is lord, and they are a slave to an evil spirit. It is their master, and it is their lord in that area of their lives. And this is the juncture where we must break down the real dilemma. Whether or not an evil spirit can possess a Christian may be the wrong question. Instead, the more important question is: "Does an evil spirit have a Christian?" To that question, the answer is, "Absolutely, yes." And to those who would deny my position, I challenge them to give me another explanation from Scripture. If someone tells me it is not an evil spirit but just their flesh, I will challenge them to explain the "old man". Many people argue that the "old man" is Satan's kingdom in us before conversion. The problem with this position is that there is evidence that we still see Satan's kingdom at play in our lives after conversion. How can that be explained?

If we were dead to sin at conversion, why do I see sin alive in people's mortal bodies afterward? This dilemma demands an answer. How can we be saved and still do the works of evil? If someone tells me it is just their flesh, that would make them a split personality. We are not split personalities. When someone says it is just their flesh, that makes them half evil and half good, and I disagree with that position. When someone says the evil manifesting through them is just their flesh, that makes them a split personality and binds them to sin as part of their nature. I have to come out of agreement with that position because Paul also came out of agreement with that in Romans 7. He said it was not he who did it when he sinned, but the sin that dwelt within him was doing the evil. It was not even him doing it. If it was not Paul who did the evil mentioned in Romans 7, then what was doing it? He said it was *sin* that did this evil through him.

*Now if I do that I would not, it is no
more I that do it, but sin that dwelleth
in me. Romans 7:20 KJV*

So sin has to be an intelligent being dwelling in Paul that did it. There is no other conclusion mentioned in this conversation. If Paul said when he sinned, it was not him that did it, then who did it? Something within him manifested through him when he gave it permission. It was not his "conscious" or "subconscious" either. If we obey righteousness, we are servants to God. But if we follow after temptation, we become a servant of sin. As a reminder, verse 16 says, "Know ye not, that to whom ye yield yourselves servants to obey, his servants ye are to whom ye obey; whether of sin unto death, or of obedience unto righteousness?"

*Know ye not, that to whom ye yield
yourselves servants to obey, his
servants ye are to whom ye obey;
whether of sin unto death, or of
obedience unto righteousness? Romans
6:16 KJV*

In our Christian lives, we have an opportunity to serve God or the devil every day. How many of us each day have the opportunity to discern good and evil? How many of us have thoughts, impressions, feelings that come to us that we know are not of God? Do we decide whether to follow the law of God or the law of sin? Many of us find these challenges are an everyday exercise of being a Christian, weighing our decisions to make proper ones. However, some people may ignore these decisions or avoid situations that could lead them into difficult situations. It is not wise to avoid problems. As I remind Christians, "out of sight and out of mind" is not a spiritual principle. We can pretend the devil and his kingdom do not exist, but we will be deceived. We may also pretend that we are sinless in the name of whatever Scripture we want to quote, but we will also be deceived because pragmatic evidence indicates otherwise.

SLAVES TO SIN

I see many people, including Christians, who are slaves to sin. They are a slave to evil spirits of fear, anxiety, bitterness, jealousy, and envy. They do not even recognize temptation. They are so trained by these evil spirits that they act them out when they are given thoughts and feelings by the spirits. For this reason, especially concerning the unsaved, much of what I am saying is not only not good but potentially dangerous to their spirituality. What good would it do to have "discerning of spirits" for somebody who is unsaved? What good would it do to cast out an evil spirit from an unsaved person? It would eventually make their situation worse. The Bible says when an evil spirit is cast out, it wanders through a dry place looking for place of rest and, finding none, returns to its original house to see if the house is filled or empty.

> *[43]When the unclean spirit is gone out of a man, he walketh through dry places, seeking rest, and findeth none. [44]Then he saith, I will return into my house from*

*whence I came out; and when he is
come, he findeth it empty, swept, and
garnished. ⁴⁵Then goeth he, and taketh
with himself seven other spirits more
wicked than himself, and they enter in
and dwell there: and the last state of
that man is worse than the first. Even
so shall it be also unto this wicked
generation. Matthew 12:43-45 KJV*

How may an unsaved person be filled with the
Holy Spirit if they are not first born again? They
cannot. The worst thing we could do to an unsaved
person is cast out an evil spirit from them because it
would come back in bringing seven much worse than
itself and the latter state of that person would be
worse than the former state.

There is just no way to help them if they refuse
to be born again. Healing is the children's bread.
Deliverance is the children's bread.

*²²And, behold, a woman of Canaan
came out of the same coasts, and cried
unto him, saying, Have mercy on me, O
Lord, thou Son of David; my daughter is
grievously vexed with a devil. ²³But he
answered her not a word. And his
disciples came and besought him,
saying, Send her away; for she crieth
after us.*

*²⁵Then came she and worshipped him,
saying, Lord, help me. ²⁶But he answered*

and said, It is not meet to take the
children's bread, and to cast it to dogs.
²⁷And she said, Truth, Lord: yet the dogs
eat of the crumbs which fall from their
masters' table. ²⁸Then Jesus answered
and said unto her, O woman, great is
thy faith: be it unto thee even as thou
wilt. And her daughter was made whole
from that very hour. Matthew 15:22-23,
25-28 KJV

If healing is the children's bread, then what do we need to be healed of? If deliverance is the children's bread, what do we need to be delivered from? If sanctification was a finished product when we became born again, we would not need either deliverance or healing. Satan would be separated from us—his kingdom would torment the unsaved, and we would be separated from them living peacefully. If the light is over here and darkness is separate over there, why do we need to be sanctified? And if that position is true and we find ourselves struggling with evil, then are we really born again?

There is a theology in a particular denomination that says if someone backslides, they were never born again. I disagree with the position that the backsliding person was never born again. I find this position to be ridiculous. If someone sins, they were never born again? How many Christians do we know who have sinned since they were born again? Maybe we are one of them. Does that mean we are not born again? No. In the area where we fall into sin, we have come back under the dominion of Satan and his kingdom. They want to be our lord and make us a slave to them in that area of our lives.

I believe Satan and his kingdom are interested in Christians — ignorant Christians. They are interested in all flesh and humanity. They need us. They are spiritual parasites and need us as a method of expression in the physical world. And when they are not in human beings manifesting their evil nature, they are in torment. When they are in a person manifesting, they are not in torment anymore. The evil spirit's peace is inverse to the person's peace. The person is in torment when the evil spirit manifests in their life. When the evil spirit is cast out, the person is at peace, and the evil spirit is in torment. Who needs to be at peace, the evil spirit or the human? Who needs to be in torment?

And so when the evil spirit is cast out, it goes into a dry place looking for a place of rest and finds none. Why? It is at unrest because it needs to manifest itself by its nature. Many people in prison for murder are the victims of a spirit of bitterness and murder. They manifested the evil, and it is a done deed. It fulfilled its nature and the human is paying the penalty for life because of the possession of an evil spirit of bitterness. America, the prison, society, and secular psychology do not understand this reality. They are holding the man responsible, which they should; do not misunderstand me. But they do not understand the murder originated with an evil spirit. An evil spirit manifested through the person who committed murder. A spirit of murder perpetrated it, and they do not even know it. We are ignorant people in the world, but God has come to give us insights by His Word.

SERVANTS OF RIGHTEOUSNESS

Returning to Romans 6, verse 16 says, "Know ye not, that to whom ye yield yourselves servants to obey, his servants ye are to whom you obey; whether of sin unto death, or of obedience unto righteousness? But God be thanked, that ye were the servants of sin, but ye have obeyed from the heart that form of doctrine which was delivered you. Being then made free from sin, ye became the servants of righteousness."

> *[16]Know ye not, that to whom ye yield yourselves servants to obey, his servants ye are to whom ye obey; whether of sin unto death, or of obedience unto righteousness? [17]But God be thanked, that ye were the servants of sin, but ye have obeyed from the heart that form of doctrine which was delivered you. [18]Being then made free from sin, ye became the servants of righteousness. Romans 6:16-18 KJV*

Is this by application? Is this present progressive? If we are being given an opportunity to follow Father God, is it a finished work? No, but it is possible for us to become free. And this is where sanctification has its beginning. We are working out our own salvation. Remember the Scripture that mentions we are to work out our own salvation with fear and trembling?

Wherefore, my beloved, as ye have always obeyed, not as in my presence only, but now much more in my absence, work out your own salvation with fear and trembling. Philippians 2:12 KJV

Why would we need to be working out our own salvation if we did not have to address it after conversion? So why does Scripture tell us to work out our own salvation? Because we are appropriating the works of righteousness right now to establish the Kingdom of God on earth by our obedience. No longer do we have to be slaves to sin. This ministry represents freedom from slavery to sin.

ROOTS OF DISEASE

Of additional importance, we have tied sin to disease because the Bible ties sin to disease in Deuteronomy 28 and Proverbs 26:2. In Deuteronomy 28, under the verses listing the curses that come from disobedience to the Word of God, Scriptures describe what can only be understood to be physical and mental illness and disease. In verses 27 and 28 of Deuteronomy 28, it lists both physical and mental problems. My understanding of the term "emerods" is another spelling of the word *hemorrhoids*. These are certainly not a blessing, and madness describes insanity, which is certainly not a blessing.

²⁷The LORD will smite thee with the botch of Egypt, and with the emerods, and with the scab, and with the itch, whereof thou canst not be healed. ²⁸The LORD shall smite thee with madness, and blindness, and astonishment of heart: Deuteronomy 28:27-28 KJV

Moving to Proverbs 26:2, it says the curse causeless does not come. What does that mean? It means that we cannot say that it was just a coincidence that we have curses and problems in our lives.

As the bird by wandering, as the swallow by flying, so the curse causeless shall not come. Proverbs 26:2 KJV

With this in mind, it is my position that 80% of diseases today are a lack of sanctification — either in our family trees or personal lives — where we have opened the door to evil spirits to come into our lives. What are the wages of sin? Death.

For the wages of sin is death; but the gift of God is eternal life through Jesus Christ our Lord. Romans 6:23 KJV

The beginning of healing all spiritually-rooted diseases is sanctification before the living God. In the case of Multiple Chemical Sensitivity/Environmental Illness (MCS/EI), a condition with many different allergies, people have experienced freedom after they repented and were sanctified in the various areas of their lives. Many have been healed of allergies as they continued in their journey. Many of them were wandering around all over the place, searching for an answer before coming to this ministry and church. Over days, months, and years, these people started to take back their lives. They often had become progressively allergic to various things in their lives. They became allergic to one food, and then a few more, and eventually could only eat a few foods. Many people had to avoid certain scents and environments because of certain chemicals. They had become a slave to fear and allergies.

Perhaps people do not have allergies, but they may have other physical, mental, or spiritual issues for which they are seeking healing and deliverance. However, the principles are the same. We are to work out our own salvation daily. We have seen many people recover from years of bondage and sickness by applying spiritual principles. As we apply Scriptures to our lives, we are no longer a slave to sin at the level that we were in the past. Following after sin allows Satan's kingdom to have a right in our life despite the cross.

I am a servant of the Most High God. I do not want to bring people under condemnation for sin, but I want to give them a reality check. Many people do not want to be told their diseases result from sin, but I want to bring them truth in order for them to be free. I have taken time to unfold this subject to be gentle and thoughtful in presenting these difficult truths. Second Timothy 2 says, "The servant of the Lord must not strive; but be gentle unto all men, apt to teach, patient, In meekness instructing those that oppose themselves; if God peradventure will give them repentance to the acknowledging of the truth; And that they may recover themselves out of the snare of the devil, who are taken captive by him at his (the devil's) will."

> [24]And the servant of the Lord must not strive; but be gentle unto all men, apt to teach, patient, [25]In meekness instructing those that oppose themselves; if God peradventure will give them repentance to the acknowledging of the truth; [26]And that they may recover themselves out of the snare of the devil, who are taken captive by him at his will. 2 Timothy 2:24-26 KJV

IDENTITY FROM SCRIPTURE

To address identity, we need to confront some questions. Who are we? Where did we come from? What is our name? Where are we going? My job, as a servant of God, is to give humanity back to God the way He wanted them from the foundation of the world, and that requires removing facets of Satan's kingdom in their lives. The degree that can be accomplished is to the degree that we are living by faith. And it will not happen overnight. There are certain Biblical principles we learn to apply over time.

Many times people may not be healed automatically. If someone is unraveling a mess of their generations and personal life, they do not necessarily go from "point A to point Z" quickly. And some people have thought like the devil in certain areas of their lives for many years. If those aspects of their personality and mind were immediately removed, they might be almost a vegetable because it would feel like much of their mindset was removed.

So what do we do? We fill up people with their identity by teaching them who they are from the Scriptures. Whom did God create from the foundation of the world? Why are they here? Are they here just taking up space, drifting through life? God is not into the "space-taking" business. When Jesus came from heaven, He did not come here to take up space. He came to this planet to destroy the works of the devil. He came to heal those who were oppressed by the devil. He came to establish the Kingdom of God in righteousness. He came to get us straightened out spiritually on the inside. He came here to fix us on the inside so that the rest of us could be fixed, including our souls/minds and bodies. I become excited every time I bump into people God has healed through our ministry. These testimonies make ministry worth it.

I used to say this about our Pastor, Anita Hill: if God raised me up just for her to be healed and become healthy spiritually, I have succeeded in the call on my life—from 55 years of tormented hell to a functional part of mankind in the Body of Christ. She came out of hell, and God restored her to His glory. She has served for long hours and asked for nothing in return. She has become a "mother in the Lord".

However, I had to be honest with her to be free, and I need to be honest with others as well. The Bible says, "Open rebuke is better than secret love."

Open rebuke is better than secret love.
Proverbs 27:5 KJV

Should I tell people a lie to make them feel better? Should I tickle their ears? If I lied, they would not respect me. People must ask themselves: do they want to be a slave to sin? Do they want to be a slave to fear? Do they want to be a slave to torment? Do they want to be a slave to anxiety? Do they be a slave to self-hatred? It is important to ask these questions and consider them when we are presented with daily situations that require a choice. I do not want to be a slave to sin and these spirits.

Chapter 9: According to the Word

THE FOUNDATION IS RELATIONSHIP

We must be awake spiritually. Many Christians are just walking through life spiritually blind. They are going to heaven, but they are missing something. The Bible has promises of heaven. It has promises of eternal life. It has promises of the Millennium and the New Heavens and New Earth, but most of the Bible has to do with the people on this planet, alive on it, and it helps them to establish the Kingdom of God in their hearts every day. It is a very pragmatic book that brings spirituality into our everyday, real-life situations.

There is nothing esoteric about these simple principles. It has basic principles to help us love the Lord our God with all of our heart, all of our soul, and all of our might. It teaches us to accept ourselves to get out of this garbage called self-condemnation, guilt, self-hatred, and lack of self-esteem so we can get on with loving our brothers as we love ourselves. The foundation of all health is *relationship*. The foundation of all disease is a breakup in relationship with either God, ourselves, or someone else. The beginning of all healing involves reconciliation with God, making peace with ourselves, and making peace with others. Whether they make peace with us or not does not make any difference. Someone has to get spiritual here, and who should be the first one to get spiritual? Other people? If we wait for unrenewed, unsaved people to change, we will be left waiting. It is time for us to choose to be spiritual despite what others have done to us.

Do we have to dress up in our robes of righteousness because we are being forced to? No. It is because of our desire and choice to follow God. It is Father God's will, and we have chosen to follow Him as His sons and daughters. That is His nature, and that is our nature. My nature is to serve Father God and humanity. I am a servant. Sometimes aspects of God's nature are ingrained in people's hearts because of the way He created them. Even before I came to the Lord, I was a good servant. I have worked with companies in the past, and they did not have to worry about my conduct — they did not have to babysit or lead me by the hand. I just took instruction and did what I had to do for them. I served and did not cause trouble. I did not cause division. I did not backbite, nor did I put down my boss. I built up these companies. I built up whomever I served.

If we are not under authority, we will never be an authority as far as God is concerned. I learned a long time ago to be under authority. That may be an oppressive word to some people because they have been under oppressive masters, family members, fathers, mothers, pastors, or teachers. But the Word of God covers that too. Even if we work in a job with a very lousy, demonized boss, we are not working for him anyway. The Word says we are working for the Lord. It is easy to serve somebody who is nice to us, but the true test of our spirituality, according to Scripture, is how we will work for somebody who is not nice to us.

22 Servants, obey in all things your masters according to the flesh; not with eyeservice, as menpleasers; but in singleness of heart, fearing God; 23 And whatsoever ye do, do it heartily, as to the Lord, and not unto men; 24 Knowing that of the Lord ye shall receive the reward of the inheritance: for ye serve the Lord Christ. Colossians 3:22-24 KJV

Naturally, we always want people to be nice to us, and then we will be spiritual with them. However, according to Scripture, the true test of our spirituality is what we are going to do when people are not nice to us. Perhaps the way we usually behave when we are exposed to people who are unrenewed and unspiritual is we become unspiritual with them — now we have a real problem. When I am around evil people, I have to choose not to react to their evil. We need to have a change of perspective. Our responses need to be according to the Word of God and not because we fall into the traps of demonic emotions. We need to operate according to Biblical knowledge.

GREATER GRACE

We teach two graces in this ministry — sustaining grace and a greater grace. We teach the sustaining grace as sufficient in times of our troubles. But we do not just stop there. We go on and teach the greater grace. His sustaining grace is His absolute grace and mercy for us in our condition when we struggle, but His greater grace replaces His sustaining grace. And the greater grace is to His absolute glory. The sustaining grace is to His glory, too; do not misunderstand me. But the greater grace is to His absolute glory because when we do not have a problem, there is a greater glory than having a problem. He does not just want to rescue us when times are tough. He also wants us to grow up spiritually and prepare us to overcome challenges in the future. There is a place for moments when we need help, but there is also a place for maturing in God as He purifies us of sin so we can withstand troubles coming our way. He does not just want us to survive—He wants us to thrive.

I am establishing a firm position on our true identities by exposing certain aspects of our thinking that may not even be us. Hopefully, my words resonate and perhaps remind people of certain observations they have made over their lifetimes. We have become so one with the enemy in our thinking that it is almost impossible to believe God today. We are living in a physical world, and the enemy comes at us in the physical dimension. Even though he is a spirit being, he knows where to get us right where it hurts. We are not entirely a physical being, but we are, in part, a physical being. We are a spirit being, and we need to stay in the Spirit no matter what is going on in our lives. It does not matter what kind of sandstorms are blowing.

In this respect, our "spirit man" is immune to the physical world and all of its problems. When we have pain in our body, our spirit man does not have pain. We feel it and sense it physiologically and psychologically, but our spirit man does not know pain. That is why the Bible says the spirit of man shall sustain him in his infirmity.

> *The spirit of a man will sustain his infirmity; but a wounded spirit who can bear? Proverbs 18:14 KJV*

What does this verse mean? It means in the midst of our battle or infirmity, our spirit can be as strong as if we never had a problem. We should be in the Spirit all the time in our inner man. How do we think the Apostle Paul went to 40 stripes twice save one, went into perils, nakedness, famine, and other trials and tribulations? It would have been easier for him to stay a Pharisee and just teach in the temple as a way of life. What took Christ to the cross for us? What does it take to be a martyr of the Christian faith? What took them there? Their spirit man was immune to the devil and everything this world has to offer. They remained in the Spirit, regardless of what was happening to them, understanding that they would be resurrected one day anyway.

What is the worst thing that can happen to us? We would die and go to heaven. So what is our problem? When we are busy trying to save our lives, we are continually losing them. Why not lose our lives so we can save them? We are hanging onto the rudiments of our lives, onto the years of our generation, hoping for 80, 90, or 100 years. We are so busy hanging onto this life that we have forgotten this lifetime is not eternal. What we have accumulated in this life is temporary. I have said this 1,000 times, and I will say it 1,001 times: 100 years from now, the vicissitudes of this life will be the last thing on our minds. That is how eternal it is. God is not insensitive to the vicissitudes of our lives; in fact, He says He is touched by the feelings of our infirmities. And do not get me wrong, God is touched by our physical existence. If not, He would not have sent Jesus to help us to overcome.

For we have not an high priest which cannot be touched with the feeling of our infirmities; but was in all points tempted like as we are, yet without sin. Hebrews 4:15 KJV

A BROKEN SPIRIT

According to the Scripture I quoted earlier, a broken spirit dries up the bones.

A merry heart doeth good like a medicine: but a broken spirit drieth the bones. Proverbs 17:22 KJV

In my experience, a broken spirit is the entrance of an evil spirit. A broken spirit is the presence of an evil spirit that has become one with us spiritually and represents the tragedy of events in our lives. When I refer to "a broken spirit", that is not a physical dimension. It relates to what we feel as temptation that begins in the spirit and corresponds to emotions and thoughts in our souls/minds. When we agree to follow after temptation, it becomes our sin. Now, we have become one in our spirit and soul with the identity of an evil spirit. Our human spirit can be cohabited by evil spirits. And because we do not understand that, we become one with them and their fallen nature. This creates a fragmentation of the human spirit. The fragmentation of the human spirit involves the intrusion of another very intelligent and real entity that wants to become part of our life spiritually.

It wants to become a part of us so it can manifest itself by its fallen nature. In that way, we become one with it. That is why Hebrews 4:12-13 is so clear. It says the Word of God is quick and powerful, sharper than a two-edged sword, is able to penetrate even to the joint and marrow (there is the physiology of man), and is a discerner of the thoughts and the intents of the heart.

> *12For the word of God is quick, and powerful, and sharper than any twoedged sword, piercing even to the dividing asunder of soul and spirit, and of the joints and marrow, and is a discerner of the thoughts and intents of the heart. 13Neither is there any creature that is not manifest in his sight: but all things are naked and opened unto the*

eyes of him with whom we have to do.
Hebrews 4:12-13 KJV

So what is in our human spirit? Thoughts and intents. Not just our psychology, not just our psyche. That word *psyche* is part of the term *psychology* and means the soul—the psyche of man, the soul of man. We could accurately call it "soul-ology" to understand the point of the term psychology. It is the study of the soul or mind.

I want to draw together a few subjects. Hebrews 4:12 says that the Word of God is quick and powerful and is a discerner of the thoughts and intents of the heart. We are not entirely focused on the psyche of humanity; we are focused on the spirit of man. I quoted earlier that as a man thinks in his heart, so is he.

For as he thinketh in his heart, so is he:
Eat and drink, saith he to thee; but his
heart is not with thee. Proverbs 23:7
KJV

As I understand it, the heart is not the soul but the spirit. Mark 7 says, "For from within, out of the heart of men, proceed evil thoughts."

For from within, out of the heart of
men, proceed evil thoughts, adulteries,
fornications, murders, Mark 7:21 KJV

It is out of the *heart* of man—not out of the soul or the psyche. Everyone is so busy chasing the psychology of man, and they do not realize the core problem is internal and spiritual. Not many people, even Christian ministers, understand the human spirit or the intrusion of demonic forces into mankind. They are so busy chasing this invisible force that they do not even know what they are talking about.

Now, there does seem to be some confusion in Christianity about a "broken spirit" versus having a "broken and contrite spirit" before God. In this case, it requires contextual understanding. As an example, I examined the word *fear* in the Bible. Specifically, I addressed the "fear of God." Many people believe they are supposed to be afraid of God. However, we found that in the Hebrew language alone, there are 14 different, distinct words that are translated into English term *fear*. In the Greek, there are seven words translated into *fear*. So which one do we want to use? When we did a word study of the *fear of the Lord* it meant reverential respect or moral reverence. Returning to the concepts of a broken heart from injury versus a humble and contrite heart — the difference is found in that a humble and contrite heart is soft and open before God. This broken spirit is one that is humble before the living God.

> *The sacrifices of God are a broken spirit:*
> *a broken and a contrite heart, O God,*
> *thou wilt not despise. Psalm 51:17 KJV*

> *For thus saith the high and lofty One*
> *that inhabiteth eternity, whose name is*

Holy; I dwell in the high and holy place,
with him also that is of a contrite and
humble spirit, to revive the spirit of the
humble, and to revive the heart of the
contrite ones. Isaiah 57:15 KJV

To understand a broken spirit in the negative context, it is my position that it is a result of injury or trauma. This is worlds apart from a contrite spirit. The main question is: how did the injury occur? Does not all injury, both spirit and soul, involve some physical event or ongoing traumas? Yes and no. At its core, it is not physical at all. A person may have been beaten by someone and physically abused, and there would be injury to their physical body. However, behind the physical abuse was something spiritual. What was it? Thought. Someone was tempted by a thought to inflict pain upon another person, and that temptation is what brought the physical abuse.

The main spiritual evidence I find when a person has a broken spirit is the words they use to describe abuse. When a person says, "Well, they hurt me," or, "I am really hurt." When I find the word *hurt* being used, I find bitterness. It has developed or is developing in their thoughts and memories. In part, our existence is comprised of the physiological functioning of our temple, as in our body, which houses our soul and spirit. However, the rest of our existence involves feelings, emotions, thoughts, concepts, precepts, ideologies, doctrines, insights, intuition, and our conscience. The latter part of our existence, apart from our physicality, has to do with words or feelings representing words and ideas. Every bit of our existence is wrapped up in conceptual thinking. Either we have good thinking or we have "stinking thinking," known as bad ideas or somewhere in-between. And this is our battleground. For this reason, we need the Word of God to lead us into all truth and out of the captivity of sin.

THE LORD GOD REVELATION

It is amazing that Jesus Christ is the Word of God. What does that mean? He represented the spoken thoughts of Father God. The Father did not speak them Himself. He sent the Word of God to speak to humanity. The God of the Old Testament is Jesus Christ in his pre-incarnate state. The member of the Godhead who created all things was Jesus Christ. He was not Jesus Christ at that time. Jesus is His earthly name, but before He came in the flesh and became one of us, He was God the Word.

While this teaching is on identity and not the one I have done on the LORD God Revelation, I want to give some information based upon that teaching to help identify the Godhead. In the Old Testament, Jesus was known as Yehovah Elohim. In the Hebrew this is "YHWH," the sacred name. The tetragrammaton with the vowel points added is transliterated as Yehovah, also translated to Jehovah, otherwise known as all capital letters "LORD" in the Old Testament. When we see "LORD God" written with all capitals in "LORD" and a capital "G" and all lowercase letters "God," this is God the Word, the second member of the Godhead, in the King James Version of the Bible. The King James Version is an English translation of the Hebrew Masoretic text. Not only is this term a combination of capitalization and lowercase, but is the translation of two Hebrew words. "LORD" phonetically is spelled Yehovah, and "God" is Elohim.

It is my position that the translators of the King James Bible used capitalization and lowercase to delineate two members of the Godhead translated from Hebrew. LORD God, or God the Word, is the authority over creation—therefore "LORD" is entirely capitalized. However, in terms of the Godhead, He is in submission to Father God. He said the Father and He were one because they are unified in the Godhead.

I and my Father are one. John 10:30

There are three members, but as Jesus said, "my Father is greater than I."

> *Ye have heard how I said unto you, I go away, and come again unto you. If ye loved me, ye would rejoice, because I said, I go unto the Father: for my Father is greater than I. John 14:28 KJV*

In the capitalization of "God" in the translation of the Hebrew Scriptures, "LORD God," or God the Word, is not the *head* of the Godhead, and therefore it is a capital "G" with the rest as lowercase. In creation, it pleased the Father that all things should be put under the authority of Jesus Christ, the Creator.

Therefore, in the capitalization of Father God in the Old Testament, it is "Lord GOD." He gave Jesus preeminence as "LORD"; therefore, it is capital "L" with the rest lowercase—Lord. But in terms of the Godhead, He is the One who has dictated His or the "Father's will" for all of creation; therefore, He is referred to as all capital letters "GOD". So even in the distinction of the capitalization in the translation of Hebrew into English, the Godhead is clearly in the Old Testament Scripture. From the translation of the Hebrew, "Lord" is the term Adonay, and "GOD" is Yehovih.

To understand how I came to this conclusion, look at Isaiah 48:16-17.

> [16]*Come ye near unto me, hear ye this; I have not spoken in secret from the beginning; from the time that it was, there am I: and now the Lord GOD, and his Spirit, hath sent me.* [17]*Thus saith the LORD, thy Redeemer, the Holy One of Israel; I am the LORD thy God which teacheth thee to profit, which leadeth thee by the way that thou shouldest go.*
> *Isaiah 48:16-17*

In verse 16, the Lord GOD is Father God or Adonai Yehovih. He is the One who sent Jesus to this planet. Jesus did not send Himself, but the Father gave us Jesus.

> *For God so loved the world, that he gave his only begotten Son, that*

whosoever believeth in him should not perish, but have everlasting life. John 3:16 KJV

In verse 17, who is the Redeemer? It is Jesus or God the Word, known in this Scripture as LORD God or Yehovah Elohim. I have found these terms to be consistent throughout the Old Testament Hebrew when "LORD God" and "Lord GOD" are used — they consistently refer to God the Word and Father God. However, this insight is not found in the New Testament as it is only in Hebrew and not Greek.

BIBLICAL ERROR

Newer English Bible translations are not translated from the Hebrew Masoretic text. They are translated from the Greek Septuagint. The problem with a Greek versus a Hebrew Old Testament foundation is the lack of these specific naming conventions because of the different languages. Without a Hebrew foundation, the Godhead revelation in the Old Testament is lost forever. I cannot teach a Jew about the Godhead from any other translation if they have a Greek Old Testament foundation. Only the King James Version matches the traditional Orthodox Hebrew Scriptures that have been around since the time of Moses. The Scriptures from Genesis to Malachi that we have today in Orthodox Judaism are the same Scriptures from the times of Christ and Moses.

One thing I have observed about the Jews is that they have meticulously preserved the Torah, the Writings, and the Prophets. And all the Gentiles of America and the world have said, "We do not like it. We will just rewrite the Bible the way we want to." From my own studies, I have found that the NIV (New International Version) has 38,000 direct translation errors between the Old and New Testament—30,000 in the Old and 8,000 in the New. If someone wants to start retranslating the Bible and getting it back correct, that would be a good place to start. I would not bother with it anymore. And while I am focused on the topic of translations, for those who have been taught the NIV is easier to read because it does not contain "thee" and "thou" and other archaic words, I have only found 300 archaic words in the entire King James Version. In the Old and New Testament, there are only 300, which could have been footnoted.

For the life of me, I do not see why 38,000 errors are a good replacement for 300 archaic words. If someone has said it is easier to read, they bought a lie by publishers selling them a new Bible to make money. The NIV and the King James Version were subjected to international testing standards for education in secular schools—colleges, universities, and public schools. There is an international testing standard to determine the reading level of a text. If someone wrote a book for children, they would subject the book to this international testing standard to determine which grade level would be appropriate for reading comprehension.

When these Bible translations were subjected to this international standard of testing of readability and grade level, it took a 5.3-grade level to read and understand the NIV, but only a 4.3 to read and understand the King James. Almost one whole grade level is required to understand and read the NIV over the King James, and that is based on international testing. I have often said I would produce another Bible if I had time. I would take the King James, and I would not tamper with it whatsoever. And when we have archaic words, I would footnote them, take out "thee" and "thou" without tampering with the manuscript, and call it the Wright Bible.

Supposedly the New King James has done that, but we have bought another lie. The New King James is not another translation of the Old King James; it is a mixture of the King James and modern translations. For instance, "the Comforter," which is the Holy Spirit, is translated as "the Helper" in the New King James Version. There is a difference between the Greek word that is translated into "Comforter" and one that is translated into "Helper." In two different Scriptures in the King James Version, these words appear—but they are not the same Greek word.

So that we may boldly say, The Lord is my helper, and I will not fear what man shall do unto me. Hebrews 13:6 KJV

Nevertheless I tell you the truth; It is expedient for you that I go away: for if I

*go not away, the Comforter will not
come unto you; but if I depart, I will
send him unto you. John 16:7 KJV*

The term *helper* is Greek 998 in the Strong's
Concordance, and it means "succorer" or "assistance
in time of distress". That term makes sense for the
translation of *helper*. The term *comforter* is Greek 3875.
It is defined as "consoler", and console can be defined
as "comfort". Therefore, the term *comforter* is an
accurate translation. We cannot use terms generically
and interchangeably. The King James Version is not
perfect; however, they thoughtfully used terms to
translate the Scriptures into English. The Holy Spirit
is my Comforter. He may be my Helper too, but He is
first my Comforter. I love that term. I love the way it
feels.

THE GOSPELS AND THE BOOK OF ACTS

At this point, it is important to bring these
various subjects into focus. The New Testament can
be broken down into four basic parts: the Gospels, the
Book of Acts, the Epistles, and it concludes with the
Book of Revelation. Understanding the lives of the
people who lived during the writing of the New
Testament is very important, as were the lives of
those during the Old Testament. However,
presuming that contextualizing the past removes their
relevance to today is a dangerous position.

Among the different types of denominations in
America, a large sect of Christianity believes that

healing and the miracles of God passed away with the Apostles; they are known as dispensationalists. In other words, they believe the miracles of God had a place in history and have since passed away. They believe God raised the dead, healed the sick, and did miracles in the entire Old Testament—He did it in the days of Christ, and He did it in the days of the Apostles. However, for the past 2,000 years, they believe healing and deliverance are not part of the atonement unless God sovereignly involves Himself because He decides to arbitrarily.

Many of their positional statements are not backed by Scripture. In fact, many of these ideologies are not founded by Scripture. They are the constructs and concepts of men's minds. They reason that because there is not an emphasis on healing and deliverance beginning in the Book of Romans, it ceased Scripturally. They further reason that if healing of disease and casting out of evil spirits were important, we would find it in Romans through the Book of Jude. They take this position because there seems to be an absence and lack of emphasis in the writings of Paul. I want to submit my position on Scripture and how I see the structure of the New Testament. Matthew, Mark, Luke, and John are the acts of Christ. The acts of Christ include the coming of Christ, His death and resurrection, and the acts of Christ along with the acts of the twelve who served Him, and the acts of the seventy whom He appointed. The Gospels are the acts of Christ.

The Book of Acts is the continuum of Christ's ministry as set forth by men, not personally by Christ. With the oversight of Christ from heaven as the work of the Holy Spirit, the Early Church continued the works of Christ. This was so that the words of Christ found in the Scriptures could be fulfilled when He said, "The works that I do shall he do also; and greater works than these shall he do; because I go unto my Father."

> *Verily, verily, I say unto you, He that believeth on me, the works that I do shall he do also; and greater works than these shall he do; because I go unto my Father. John 14:12 KJV*

And so we have the Book of Acts or the acts of the First Century Church. I believe the Book of Acts is still being written—not on earth, but in heaven; there is a running account of what is happening. I fully intend to have a chapter of my life in that great book of eternity. I am doing the acts of the Church today. I expect that there will be tens of thousands of people in the New Testament Church in the past 2,000 years who will be found in the "great acts of the Church" book that is still being written in heaven. When we rule as Kings and Priests coming out of the Tribulation period, all the natural men of eternity will need to be taught history. The Bible is the history of God's people. I believe the past 2,000 years will also be recorded for posterity in the eons of time. I suspect we will find interesting people in those pages who believed God and went about serving Him in their generations by faith—not because they had to, not because they were forced to, but just because they loved God and believed Him. And so we have the Book of Acts, which describes the acts of the Apostles and the acts of the Early Church to demonstrate the Kingdom of God's authority over the kingdom of the devil regardless of the power of sin. It demonstrates God's love and the supremacy of the Kingdom of God over the kingdom of the devil in spite of sin so that we may see God's heart and His power over evil. That is the greater grace: God's sovereign fulfillment of the Scriptures that said He would have mercy on whom He would have mercy, based upon His own decision.

> *Therefore hath he mercy on whom he will have mercy, and whom he will he hardeneth. Romans 9:18 KJV*

We need to make sure we do not limit God in our thinking. Father God can heal and deliver us regardless of where we are at in life. It is His will, and He is capable of intervening regardless of how unworthy the devil believes we are of His mercy.

THE EPISTLES

Now, we have moved past the acts of the Apostles and the acts of the Church to the Epistles. Beginning in Romans 1, there is a massive statement on the subject of sin and its nature. Then it says in Hebrews 4:12: "For the word of God is quick, and powerful, and sharper than any twoedged sword, piercing even to the diving asunder of soul and spirit, and of the joints and marrow, and is a discerner of the thoughts and intents of the heart." Then verse 13 says, "Neither is there any creature that is not made manifest in his sight: but all things are naked and opened unto the eye of him with whom we have to do."

> [12]For the word of God is quick, and powerful, and sharper than any twoedged sword, piercing even to the dividing asunder of soul and spirit, and of the joints and marrow, and is a discerner of the thoughts and intents of the heart. [13]Neither is there any creature that is not manifest in his sight: but all things are naked and opened unto the eyes of him with whom we have to do. Hebrews 4:12-13 KJV

What is naked and open before God? Creatures. What creatures? My position on that Scripture is that those are principalities and powers, the rulers of the darkness of this world, spiritual wickedness in high places otherwise known as evil spirits, and the entire kingdom of the second heaven. I know that kingdom; I am at war with it all the time. I fight an invisible enemy, but I see him just as clearly as if I could see him with my physical eyes — that is part of spiritual discernment.

How can we have discernment of spirits if we cannot identify the spirits? The Church is so busy attempting to fight the devil personally that they forgot we are fighting his kingdom. So who are we fighting against? Satan is not omnipresent. Who are we fighting? Who are we warring against? Why do we need the Word of God to separate the soul from the spirit? Why do creatures need to be made manifest? As an example of identifying a spirit, I consider adultery to be an evil spirit. I consider lust to be an evil spirit. I consider envy and jealousy to be evil spirits. I consider fear to be an evil spirit. I consider rage and anger to be evil spirits, not emotions, which have become ingrained within our hearts. We have become one with them in our thinking—both at a spirit level and then as a soulish part of our identity. That is why the Word of God has to separate the spirit from the soul to bring back some sanity to our thinking.

Someone may believe being bitter is a way of life. They may believe it is just the way they are. No, they have a devil. That statement makes people "nervous and jerky" because they have a fear of evil. Shame on them; how dare they be afraid of the devil! How dare they be afraid of evil! When we are afraid of evil, we are enthroning and enshrining Satan as god of the world all over again. When we yield our minds to the aspects of Satan's nature through his kingdom in us, we are enthroning him in our hearts. Paul cut through this subject in Romans 6: whomever we yield ourselves to is our master, and we are its slave. And we are following another law.

Know ye not, that to whom ye yield
yourselves servants to obey, his

servants ye are to whom ye obey;
whether of sin unto death, or of
obedience unto righteousness? Romans
6:16 KJV

Remember Romans 7? We are following another law; it is the word of Satan versus the Word of God. Satan does not have a bible. He is too chicken to write one. So he writes on the "tables of our hearts" through thoughts of temptation, and we listen to him.

[21]I find then a law, that, when I would do good, evil is present with me. [22]For I delight in the law of God after the inward man: [23]But I see another law in my members, warring against the law of my mind, and bringing me into captivity to the law of sin which is in my members. Romans 7:22-23 KJV

THE MIND OF CHRIST

God is not scared and deceptive like Satan. He came and wrote it on pages by the Holy Spirit by holy prophets, men of old, who wrote as the Holy Ghost moved on them to establish the living Word of God in writing.

For the prophecy came not in old time by the will of man: but holy men of God spake as they were moved by the Holy Ghost. 2 Peter 1:21 KJV

It is time to tear apart Satan's kingdom. We need to take his thoughts and his word, and take them and hold them to the light of Scripture. The true test of our spirituality, when it comes to warfare, is our ability to hold good and evil. With evil in one hand and good in the other, scrutinize both to see which is of God and which is not—all the time. That is what 2 Corinthians 10:5 is all about. It is about holding every thought in captivity, casting out every imagination, everything that would exalt itself against the knowledge of God. What is the knowledge of God? We have been told we have the mind of Christ. Do we put on the mind of Christ when we feel like it? So, what is the mind of Christ? He is the Word.

Casting down imaginations, and every high thing that exalteth itself against the knowledge of God, and bringing into captivity every thought to the obedience of Christ; 2 Corinthians 10:4 KJV

For who hath known the mind of the Lord, that he may instruct him? but we have the mind of Christ. 1 Corinthians 2:16 KJV

The Word of God is a full extension of the will of Father God. So, when we have the mind of Christ, we have the mind of the Father. Why do I know that? Because Jesus said it. He told us that He only said what He heard the Father saying.

Then said Jesus unto them, When ye have lifted up the Son of man, then shall

ye know that I am he, and that I do
nothing of myself; but as my Father
hath taught me, I speak these things.
John 8:28 KJV

When Jesus spoke, He represented Father God.
Therefore, Jesus' words represented the Father's
words. So, what would the Father say to us? Blessed
are the merciful, for they shall obtain mercy. Forgive
your brother. Love the Lord your God with all your
heart, all your soul, and all your might. Love your
neighbor as yourself.

Blessed are the merciful: for they shall obtain
mercy. Matthew 5:7 KJV
And when ye stand praying, forgive, if
ye have ought against any: that your
Father also which is in heaven may
forgive you your trespasses. Mark 11:25
KJV

And he answering said, Thou shalt love
the Lord thy God with all thy heart, and
with all thy soul, and with all thy
strength, and with all thy mind; and thy
neighbour as thyself. Luke 10:27 KJV

When Jesus started His ministry, He did not
begin with miracles and teaching. He started in
Matthew 5 with the Sermon on the Mount—the
Beatitudes. And every bit of the Beatitudes deals with
the relationship of God with man. What does Satan
come to do at a core level? He comes to destroy
relationships between God and man. Wars

throughout humanity, family breakups, and insanity all result from a breakdown in this relationship.

THE LORD'S RIGHTEOUSNESS

Now, remember that Hebrews 4:13 says that every creature is made manifest in His sight?

Neither is there any creature that is not manifest in his sight: but all things are naked and opened unto the eyes of him with whom we have to do. Hebrews 4:13 KJV

In order to fight Satan's scheme, we must discern how he sneaks into our lives. Romans 1:18 says, "For the wrath of God is revealed from heaven against all ungodliness and unrighteousness of men, who hold the truth in unrighteousness."

For the wrath of God is revealed from heaven against all ungodliness and unrighteousness of men, who hold the truth in unrighteousness; Romans 1:18 KJV

What does "hold the truth in unrighteousness" mean? It means that we may know the truth but refuse to apply it. When we do not apply the truth, what does that produce? Unrighteousness. When we know the truth and do it, what does that make us? Righteous.

For the LORD knoweth the way of the
righteous: but the way of the ungodly
shall perish. Psalm 1:6 KJV

It is righteousness — not self-righteousness, but righteousness. It is not righteousness that originates with us, but by application, the Lord's righteousness is manifested through us by choosing to follow Him. So if we know the truth that we are to forgive our brother and do forgive him, what is manifesting through us? That is righteousness. However, what is that to us if we do not forgive our brother? That is unrighteousness. And the day we do not forgive our brother, we are holding the truth in unrighteousness. I hope that brings understanding to that term so we do not "hold the truth in unrighteousness" ourselves.

THE GODHEAD

Moving on to the following verses in Romans, it says, "Because that which may be known of God is manifest in them; for God hath shewed it unto them. For the invisible things of him from the creation of the world are clearly seen, being understood by the things that are made, even his eternal power and Godhead."

19Because that which may be known of
God is manifest in them; for God hath
shewed it unto them. 20For the invisible
things of him from the creation of the
world are clearly seen, being understood
by the things that are made, even his

eternal power and Godhead; so that
they are without excuse: Romans 1:19-
20 KJV

The word, Godhead, used here is very important. I do not use the word "trinity" in my teachings. The word "trinity" is not found in Scriptures; it is a religious term that was coined by an apostate church. The Apostate Church has attempted to remove many Biblical concepts from their contexts. When a concept is removed from Biblical context, it requires an expert to decipher what is being said. As believers, we should be able to read and see it for ourselves in the Bible. The further we remove ourselves from the Bible itself, the further we are corrupted from the simplicity of Scripture.

> *[3]But I fear, lest by any means, as the serpent beguiled Eve through his subtilty, so your minds should be corrupted from the simplicity that is in Christ. [4]For if he that cometh preacheth another Jesus, whom we have not preached, or if ye receive another spirit, which ye have not received, or another gospel, which ye have not accepted, ye might well bear with him. 2 Corinthians 11:3-4 KJV*

The concept of "the trinity" is correct, but the term "trinity" is not found in Scripture. The Biblical term used in the King James Version is *Godhead*. What is the eternal Godhead? It has the same meaning as the concept of "the trinity". Please, do not misunderstand my heart; I am not splitting hairs. I am simply determined to remain Scriptural. For instance, I also do not use the word "rapture" anymore. It is not found in the Bible. However, the concept is accurate. The Biblical term is *First Resurrection*. I have asked many people, "What is the First Resurrection?" They do not have any idea. The Bible says that the people who are part of the First Resurrection are blessed, and they shall not taste the second death.

> *Blessed and holy is he that hath part in the first resurrection: on such the second death hath no power, but they shall be priests of God and of Christ, and shall reign with him a thousand years.*
> *Revelation 20:6 KJV*

So, what is the First Resurrection? It is "the rapture". So why not call it the First Resurrection? Why not use the word Godhead? This term is capitalized, by the way, in the majority text. I hope the word Godhead is capitalized in the Bibles we are reading. And what is the Godhead? It is the *echad* or unity of Deuteronomy 6:4 that reveals the plurality of the Godhead. It says, "Here, O Israel: the LORD our God is one LORD."

> *Hear, O Israel: The LORD our God is one LORD: Deuteronomy 6:4 KJV*

The word *one* is not a singular term but plural. It is *echad* or unity. The unity is not singular but a plural entity. It matches the plural language used in

Genesis 1:26 when it says, "And God said, Let us make man in our image."

And God said, Let us make man in our image, after our likeness: and let them have dominion over the fish of the sea, and over the fowl of the air, and over the cattle, and over all the earth, and over every creeping thing that creepeth upon the earth. Genesis 1:26 KJV

It also matches the Tower of Babel when the Lord said, "Let us go down, and there confound their language."

⁶And the LORD said, Behold, the people is one, and they have all one language; and this they begin to do: and now nothing will be restrained from them, which they have imagined to do. ⁷Go to, let us go down, and there confound their language, that they may not understand one another's speech. Genesis 11:6-7 KJV

As a reminder to the earlier LORD God insight, Isaiah 48:16-17 says, "And now the Lord GOD (Adonai Jehovih), and his Spirit, hath sent me." Whom did He send? Jehovah Elohim or God the Word. Separate members of the Godhead are found in the Hebrew language.

¹⁶Come ye near unto me, hear ye this; I have not spoken in secret from the beginning; from the time that it was,

there am I: and now the Lord GOD, and
his Spirit, hath sent me. ¹⁷*Thus saith the*
LORD, thy Redeemer, the Holy One of
Israel; I am the LORD thy God which
teacheth thee to profit, which leadeth
thee by the way that thou shouldest go.
Isaiah 48:16-17

The last chapter of Matthew says we should baptize in the name of the Father, the Son, and the Holy Ghost.

Go ye therefore, and teach all nations,
baptizing them in the name of the
Father, and of the Son, and of the Holy
Ghost: Matthew 28:19 KJV

And who is the Son? John told us who the Son was in John 1: "In the beginning was the Word, and the Word was with God, and the Word was God." And then it says the Word became flesh and dwelt amongst us.

In the beginning was the Word, and the
Word was with God, and the Word was
God. John 1:1 KJV

And the Word was made flesh, and
dwelt among us, (and we beheld his
glory, the glory as of the only begotten
of the Father,) full of grace and truth.
John 1:14 KJV

VAIN IMAGINATIONS

And now we have a picture of the eternal Godhead. However, even with His eternal power and Godhead, some people reject His Word. Nonetheless, as Romans 1:20-21 says, "So that they are without excuse: Because that, when they knew God, they glorified him not as God, neither were thankful; but became vain in their imaginations."

> *20 For the invisible things of him from the creation of the world are clearly seen, being understood by the things that are made, even his eternal power and Godhead; so that they are without excuse: 21Because that, when they knew God, they glorified him not as God, neither were thankful; but became vain in their imaginations, and their foolish heart was darkened. Romans 1:20-21 KJV*

What are imaginations? Thoughts. A few years ago, I saw a bumper sticker in Florida that said, "I don't forgive; I just get even." Well, what does that sticker stand for? That is a vain imagination. Imaginations are thoughts. Where do thoughts come from? Our thoughts have three sources — our own head and mental processes, the Godhead through the work of the Holy Spirit, and the devil through his evil spirits. The first, second, and third heaven have access to us. The first heaven is us. The second heaven is Satan through his spirits. The third heaven is God accessing us through the Holy Spirit.

Now, where are those thoughts coming from? Satan comes as an angel of light. How would Satan come to us as an angel of light? Would he come in here in a brilliant light and say, "I am Satan, the angel of light?" No. He comes with his own words as if it were a word from God. He sends an evil spirit of divination to speak to humans. The word divination in the Greek of the New Testament is the word *python*. The spirit of Python spoke through the Oracle of Delphi out of Greek mythology.

DIVINATION

In the days of the Apostle Paul, he cast out the spirit of divination in a young lady. In the Greek, the word *divination* is the same word as python. It is a Greek word, capitalized, meaning oracle. Does this term remind us of a certain serpent? That serpent would be Satan.

> *And the great dragon was cast out, that old serpent, called the Devil, and Satan, which deceiveth the whole world: he was cast out into the earth, and his angels were cast out with him.*
> *Revelation 12:9 KJV*

The equivalent of Python in yoga is Kundalini, and Kundalini would be divination. In fact, yoga is very dangerous to spiritual health. In the Eastern Mysticism of yoga, in the ascendancies of awakening Kundalini, he is awakened from the base of the spine. Via chakras in meditative states, he unfolds himself until he finally envelopes the brain and the head. I have dealt with people who have been possessed by this spirit, and I have cast it out. They have told me there was something on their head, with eyes looking around all the time. Years ago, a young man who had the spirit of Kundalini came to me. He was a high school student at 17 years of age, and I spoke to the spirit. He went right down on the floor, and his sternum was on the floor. His hands were up in the air, his feet were up in the air, and he slithered like a snake all over the place. I cast the spirit out of him.

I also cast the spirit of Kundalini out of someone in Houston years ago. Not only did God deliver her from the spirit of Kundalini, but God healed her of five incurable diseases. She gave her testimony of what happened during a seminar in Houston. It was my first time in Houston. Of that audience, about 50% disagreed with me and what I teach. They were a wide range of New Age and so on. Therefore, I was trying to be all things to all men, and I tried to do a very professional type of presentation.

About 45 minutes into my teaching, God spoke to me and said, "Cut the crap." We had the presentation on video and I was recorded saying, "What did You say, God?" I was in the middle of teaching and I abruptly paused to check my own head, which heaven was that thought coming from? "Cut the crap," He said. Then He continued, "You are trying to placate the enemy, and I called you here to establish my Kingdom." And, in my heart, I said, "Well, God, what do You want me to do?" He said, "I want you to immediately take on yoga and Kundalini for size." I answered, "No, God, I cannot do that. One-third of my audience are practitioners of yoga." In my heart, I heard God say, "I know, and when you take it on for size they are going to leave, and then I can get on with doing what I need to do."

I did it, and they left. They walked out en masse. One-third of that audience left within five to ten minutes. I said, "Yoga is supported by an evil spirit of divination. And if you practice it, you have it, and it needs to be cast out because it will keep you from God. It will keep you from reading your Bibles. It will take you down highways and modalities that will damn your soul." And they walked out. At that point, a regal Pakistani woman stood up in the audience, weeping. She was going to a Seventh-Day Adventist Church, but she was also going to a Buddhist temple to worship with her Buddhist husband. When I said what I said, she stood up in the middle of the audience and confessed before God and man. She stood there and confessed her sins openly and publicly.

As I stood back, right in the middle of the seminar, God spoke to my heart and said, "Because she has humbled herself before me and men, I am going to deliver her." I heard this statement in my spirit. When she finished confessing, I said, "Sister, God has spoken to me. Because you have humbled yourself before men and before God, He has told me He is going to deliver you of Kundalini. Would you come here, please?" She came and stood before me and I spoke to it in the name of the Lord Jesus Christ, and I said, "Kundalini, you foul spirit of divination, come out of her." And the spirit manifested in her. Later she told me it wanted to kill me, but it had no power. On the video, it can be seen; she shook her hands because the spirit in her manifested to try to do me damage. Five times it gestured, and it was gone.

Later in the seminar, I ministered healing to her later, and God healed her of five incurable diseases — including diabetes. It is a documented healing of diabetes. She left a totally different woman. God met her that day. If God stopped me for that one woman, it was worth it. That is the way I look at that experience. It was worth it.

Divination comes out of the second heaven. Divination will always counterfeit God and speak as if it were God speaking. Many times it will come with Scripture. Most divination, including New Age, uses Scriptures to validate its own beliefs, which are contrary to the Bible. What really boils my blood is *A Course in Miracles*. It was written by a devil through a woman who did channeling and automatic handwriting. To be clear, automatic handwriting occurs when someone does not consider what they are writing and, in an "automatic" fashion, writes whatever comes to their mind onto paper. This book is filled with Scripture. It is filled with Scripture from chapter to chapter, but no Bible references are given. The only way someone would know it is Scripture is if they knew their Bible. But those interested in *A Course in Miracles* do not read their Bibles; they are not even born again. Actually, many Christians do read *A Course in Miracles* because it sounds so right. That is until they read the chapter that says disease is an illusion and people do not have to repent for sin because sin is a negative concept and does not exist.

A Course in Miracles is an "angel of light" that has come and written it through massive spiritual plagiarism. Plagiarism is when a person writes something as if it were their own thoughts and they were the source of it. But somebody else wrote it, and they do not give them credit; that is plagiarism. The devil is the greatest plagiarist of all. Remember I taught that Satan came to Eve with the Word? He used the Word, but he twisted and added to it. That one verse he quoted was part of canon Scripture at that time. When Satan came to Jesus to tempt him, what did he use? He quoted from the Books of Deuteronomy and Psalms.

Does Satan know Deuteronomy and Psalms? Satan knows far more about the Bible than anyone reading this text. He has been a master of the Word for thousands of years. When we look at false religions and cults and all these modalities of thinking that are entirely anti-Christ or against Christ in their evil, they always use some facet of the word. One religious book takes roughly 50% of the Old Testament Scriptures. Another religious group took much of the Bible and changed and added to Scriptures to support their cultish beliefs. Another group uses the Bible but wrote other books to change their interpretation of God's Word. They are a mixture of God's Word and the mindset of Satan.

Father God created us to be spiritual. Father God is the *Father of spirits,* and our relationship to Him — and our identity — is tied to who we are spiritually according to the Word of God. Through spirits of divination, Satan will lure people away in their hunger and need to be a man or woman of God. And he will insert himself into their understanding of the Godhead and the Bible. The only sanity we have is to know the Word of God in context — not just the context of the chapter and book of the Bible itself but in the context of other Scriptures. The Bible says the Word of God will be established in the mouth (in the presence) of two or three witnesses.

> *This is the third time I am coming to you. In the mouth of two or three witnesses shall every word be established. 2 Corinthians 13:1 KJV*

When I believe I have found truth in Scripture, I look for it elsewhere in the Bible. If I think I have a revelation of Scripture, I do not jump on it quickly. I go find the confirmation somewhere else in Scripture by another writer. I have always found the confirmation somewhere so that the Word may be established out of the mouth of two or more witnesses. Looking for a witness in Scripture is a rule of thumb that I use as a minister. However, not just as a minister, but first because I am a believer. I am just like everyone else. I am a little sheep that became a shepherd, but I am still a sheep. I am no different than others. I do not teach from the standpoint of arrogant authority. I teach from the standpoint of humble application. I hope that everyone sees it that way. I am not trying to convince anyone of anything apart from the Bible. I am a teacher, and I am responsible to teach according to the Bible. At the same time, when I teach, everyone is responsible to prove it in the Bible for themselves. We must prove all things.

I have said this before, and I will say it again: it is everyone's responsibility to be like the Bereans. The Bereans received the Word with joy, went home, and made sure the preacher was correct. They checked it out and made sure it was true.

> *¹⁰And the brethren immediately sent away Paul and Silas by night unto Berea: who coming thither went into the synagogue of the Jews. ¹¹These were more noble than those in Thessalonica, in that they received the word with all readiness of mind, and searched the scriptures daily, whether those things were so. Acts 17:10-11 KJV*

Much of the Christian Church does not take time to do research in their Bibles; they are just like guppies. The guppy fish, at the surface of the fishbowl, just eat what they are given. Someone might say, "Bless God; that is the greatest revelation." Except what I have said should not be a new revelation. I am simply tapping into something that was already written long ago. It is entertaining when the Nobel Prize is given to someone for making a great scientific discovery. I laugh at the vanity of it. It already existed. If it did not first exist, they would not be able to discover it. They just tapped into a little bit of what God designed in creation and congratulated themselves. They could not have understood it at all if God had not allowed them to do so.

Verse 21 of Romans 1 says, "Because that, when they knew God, they glorified him not as God, neither were thankful; but became vain in their imaginations."

Because that, when they knew God, they glorified him not as God, neither were thankful; but became vain in their imaginations, and their foolish heart was darkened. Romans 1:21 KJV

What are imaginations? They are thoughts. I want everyone to be awake. I do not want people to be deceived by the devil. It is dangerous for their health. Satan's imaginations are dangerous for their sanity. It is dangerous for their spiritual well-being. Why do I teach the Word of God? To give people knowledge, not to puff them up with vanity and intellectual knowledge. Instead, so they may be able to discern good from evil. One of the key components of this church and ministry is the discerning of good and evil all the time. That does not mean that we are "sin conscious". People may say, "Well, Pastor Henry talks an awful lot about evil. I think he is overly concerned about sin." Somebody recently said, "I just think he has sin consciousness." If someone reads their Bible from Genesis to Revelation, 50% of it has to do with sin and evil. Do we read our Bibles? Does a lot of it have to do with evil, identifying it, and defining what is good and evil? The entire Bible is a declaration of what is good and what is evil.

THE DOCTRINE OF BALAAM

Now, I intend to deliver the punchline to the subjects I discussed earlier. Matthew, Mark, Luke, and John are the acts of Christ and the early disciples. The Book of Acts is the acts of the Apostles and the Early Church. There is a shift as the Scriptures transition into the Epistles. Beginning in Romans, we are not just dealing with a demonstration of God's sovereignty over evil; we are dealing with sanctification. When we are reading through the Book of Romans on into Jude, there are aspects dealing with prophecy, the second coming of Christ, church government, issues over legalism and grace and mercy, and intertwined in it is the heart of Father God related to concepts and topics covered in the Old Testament. However, underlying all of these topics, as we read the Epistles, there are teachings all about sanctification. Why? Because God cannot overlook and condone evil in humans. God will not give us blessings and let us keep our evil. He will care for us in the midst of our evil, and He will bless us because He is sovereign and He loves us, but He cannot allow us to stay in sin and bless us.

As a part of His nature, His way of thinking, and who He is, He will not bless us continually, long term, and let us keep our evil. We must be sanctified in order to maintain the integrity of our health—spirit, soul, and body. That is why the rest of the Bible in the New Testament does not emphasize healing and deliverance. Its emphasis is on sanctification because without sanctification, we will get sick. Without sanctification, we will not be healed (nor healthy) in most cases. Sanctification does not invalidate healing and deliverance; it gives us a foundation of ongoing freedom and growth. Without sanctification, God would be condoning evil in our lives in the name of blessing, which is the Doctrine of Balaam. The Doctrine of Balaam is in the Church now. The Doctrine of Balaam essentially states that we can sin like the devil without conscience or consequence. There is always a consequence for sin, thus the need for repentance and sanctification.

> *14But I have a few things against thee, because thou hast there them that hold the doctrine of Balaam, who taught Balac to cast a stumblingblock before the children of Israel, to eat things sacrificed unto idols, and to commit fornication.*
> *15So hast thou also them that hold the doctrine of the Nicolaitans, which thing I hate. 16Repent; or else I will come unto thee quickly, and will fight against them with the sword of my mouth.*
> *Revelation 2:14-16 KJV*

Chapter 10: Our Eternal Future

THE BOOK OF REVELATION

The Book of Revelation is the blessings of God for all of mankind for eternity, the establishment of His Kingdom, and the destruction of Satan's kingdom once and for all.

Now, I want to throw a hard curve ball. I want to give a greater overview or an "umbrella view" of Scripture. In the Book of Revelation, we read about the Millennium, the 1,000-year reign of Christ, and the New Heavens and the New Earth. Without reteaching the prophetic timeline, it is my position that coming out of the seven-year tribulation period at the end of the reign of the Antichrist, we will come into the Millennium or Millennial Reign of Christ. Coming out of the Millennium or 1,000 years, we will be at the White Throne Judgment. After the White Throne Judgment will be the New Heavens and the New Earth, and Jerusalem will come down out of heaven. That is the progression of events coming up afterward; I just gave a perspective on where we are going.

I really want to challenge everyone because I am putting my finger on the devil and evil spirits that become part of us. I am shining the light of Scripture on the sin that dwells within which Jesus taught us in Mark 7 and Paul taught us in Romans 7. There is a factor that I must insert into our hearts firmly that will challenge us. We may have iniquity and we may be in sin—and there may not even be an evil spirit involved at all. Now, we have two dimensions of sin. I want to give an example because I want sin to be defeated on both levels: spirit and soul. I want to give some Scriptural insight. It is my position that the covering cherub mentioned in Ezekiel 28 was Lucifer, who became Satan after he fell. He was perfect in all his ways from the day he was created. That is what the Scriptures state. That was, until iniquity was found in his heart.

> *14Thou art the anointed cherub that covereth; and I have set thee so: thou wast upon the holy mountain of God; thou hast walked up and down in the midst of the stones of fire. 15Thou wast perfect in thy ways from the day that thou wast created, till iniquity was found in thee. Ezekiel 28:14-15 KJV*

Did he have a devil when his heart turned against God? There was no such being at that time. There were no devils, there were no demons, and there were no fallen angels. There was no such thing. He had a "virus," so to speak. Every created being is capable of erring in thought personally, and then hanging onto that error and exalting it against the living God and what He has said. Every created being is capable of having a thought that is an aberration of what God has said, hanging onto it, and developing it against the knowledge of God. Every created being is capable of sinning. The only beings who are not capable of sinning are the Godhead.

*Let no man say when he is tempted, I
am tempted of God: for God cannot be
tempted with evil, neither tempteth he
any man: James 1:13 KJV*

All other created beings—angels, archangels,
covering cherubs—can fall away from God. Lucifer
was a covering cherub. One-third of all angels
followed Lucifer.

*And his tail drew the third part of the
stars of heaven, and did cast them to the
earth: and the dragon stood before the
woman which was ready to be
delivered, for to devour her child as
soon as it was born. Revelation 12:4
KJV*

They made a choice. They made a
decision. Iniquity was found in Lucifer's heart.
For as a man thinketh in his heart, so is he.

*For as he thinketh in his heart, so is he:
Eat and drink, saith he to thee; but his
heart is not with thee. Proverbs 23:7
KJV*

That is why it is so important to take our
thoughts and line them up with what God has said.
Divination is a very serious problem in the world
today; it is a very serious problem in the Christian
Church. I am not against the Holy Spirit whatsoever. I
am not against the gifts of the Holy Spirit whatsoever.

I operate in them myself, but I am against the counterfeit. And, I am against leadership who does not stand up and identify what is of God and what is not of God, and lead correctly. Addressing sin honestly and realizing we can still choose to disobey with or without evil spirits must be understood, even from the fall of Lucifer.

IMPLEMENT CHRIST'S KINGDOM

In the Millennium, Satan will be bound for 1,000 years. However, evil spirits will not also be bound. We, the Church, as Kings and Priests, shall rule with a rod of iron until we have brought all enemies of Christ to defeat. The last of which is death. That is during the Millennium. What is death in this case? It is a spirit of death.

> *²⁵For he must reign, till he hath put all enemies under his feet. ²⁶The last enemy that shall be destroyed is death. 1 Corinthians 15:25-26 KJV*

In the Millennium, we will be new creatures — not by faith but living in the actuality of glorified bodies. We will be able to operate in the spiritual and physical dimensions at the speed of thought, just as Christ did as He showed us after His resurrection. He could appear in a room and never walk through the door.

> *Then the same day at evening, being the first day of the week, when the doors*

were shut where the disciples were
assembled for fear of the Jews, came
Jesus and stood in the midst, and saith
unto them, Peace be unto you. John
20:19 KJV

It is my position that we will be able to see into
the spiritual dimension and see every demon of hell
as we look at people right now. Evil spirits are in
every single human on the face of the earth. Are we
ready for this type of warfare? Are we ready to lead
mankind into righteousness? Are we ready to lead
mankind in the Millennium across the face of this
earth? Are we willing to challenge them with this
knowledge and insight to reveal what has corrupted
the nations and our families for generations? Are we
ready to enter into that kind of discernment? I am. I
am doing it now by faith. How much easier will it be
on that day when I can see these spiritual critters face
to face rather than discern by what manifests out of
humans? I will be able to say, "Hey, spirit of fear,
how are you doing today? What are you doing here?"

In the Millennium, everything must be
defeated on this planet, and natural man must be
prepared to deal with thoughts that oppose Father
God's will. Natural man, and nations coming out of
the present time, must address the philosophies and
world religions they have followed. We also have
nations coming out of New Age beliefs. There is a
combination of ideas and beliefs across the face of this
earth. Our job, as Kings and Priests, will be to

implement Christ's Kingdom and the knowledge of the Lord until the world is in subjection to Christ.

> ²⁷*For he hath put all things under his feet. But when he saith all things are put under him, it is manifest that he is excepted, which did put all things under him.* ²⁸*And when all things shall be subdued unto him, then shall the Son also himself be subject unto him that put all things under him, that God may be all in all. 1 Corinthians 15:27-28 KJV*

Who will bring the people to be subjected unto Christ? We will. We might as well start practicing now. We might as well start demonstrating that authority now. Eternity does not begin in the First Resurrection—we are living in eternity right now. And everything we are, whoever we are, and whatever we are now is making an eternal difference. When we die, we do not begin to exist. Who we are now will carry on into the future. Part of our identity right now requires implementing the vision of Father God for our eternal future. If we do not prepare to follow Him now, how will we implement His will when we are able to clearly see His vision in the future?

> *For now we see through a glass, darkly; but then face to face: now I know in part; but then shall I know even as also I am known. 1 Corinthians 13:12 KJV*

I do not believe in retirement in the Kingdom of God. I do not believe in planned obsolescence. Our human spirit does not get old, and the Holy Ghost does not get old in it. If we buy into the spirit of death that comes with aging along with euthanasia, and the retirement business built into the fabric of modern society, we have just opened our hearts to becoming obsolete ourselves. I believe God's people should walk into eternity. When we have finished the call of God on our lives in our generation, we will know it is time to lay down our spirits and go on to the third heaven with Father God to await the First Resurrection.

For now, we just keep on moving regardless of our age. Until that day comes, do not become a vegetable. This planet needs us.

WILL WE FOLLOW GOD?

It is important to understand our choices and decisions. Lucifer did not have a devil. He had a thought, and it felt good to him. He might have said, "I am tired of leading creation in praise and worship. I am tired of being a covering cherub. I want Father God's job and throne instead." What will we choose to do? As Kings and Priests in the Millennium, we will not have an evil spirit within us. But that does not mean we will not have the ability to choose to rebel against God. If Lucifer was capable of rebellion, we are no less capable of rebellion, either.

We are called after the Order of Melchizedek. We are all after the Order of Melchizedek through Christ.

> *The LORD hath sworn, and will not repent, Thou art a priest for ever after the order of Melchizedek. Psalm 110:4 KJV*

I firmly believe that one day in eternity, each of us will have a planet to rule over, just like Lucifer. In the expansion and the population explosion of natural humans over millions of years of eternity, I can see planets continually filled with people. So the question for us, as future Kings and Priests, is who does God have on His hands? Another Lucifer? That is why our hearts are being tried right now. Will we obey the Word of God despite Satan's kingdom tempting us to rebel? If God gave me a planet of five million people, what would I do with them? Would I lead them into sedition against the living God and become like a "god" to them, or will I to serve the living God and leave them to Him? If God cannot trust me now, He cannot trust me in the future. The Bible says we will be known as we are known now.

> *For now we see through a glass, darkly; but then face to face: now I know in part; but then shall I know even as also I am known. 1 Corinthians 13:12 KJV*

We need to appropriate our identities in Christ. We need to quit listening to the devil, the decadence and death of mankind, and humanistic wisdom. We need to have an eternal picture of who we are. I have a picture of who I am that is still developing as I learn from the Word of God. It is still developing, but I like it. In the Millennium, I would be happy to have a little chapel of about 15, 20, or 30 people coming and going; I would teach them about the living God. In my prayer to Father God, I have said, "Just give them to me, Lord. I will teach them. Just give them to me, God, I would teach them everything that You taught me about Yourself."

Angels had thoughts of their own as well. When Lucifer tempted them, they made poor decisions. They followed the thought of another being. One-third of them fell. It is my position that there was creation on this planet before Adam and Eve; these beings were judged. I believe this earth was populated before the Ice Age roughly 13,000 years ago. I have an entire teaching on the subject of Spirit World Realities, so I do not want to expand upon this subject and detract from this teaching. My point is that the covering cherub, Lucifer, lead creation in rebellion against Father God. I refer to it as the age that was ruled by angels. In contrast, this age is ruled by Jesus Christ. The age to come will be ruled by Jesus Christ and the saints forever. However, to remain on point, it is important to return to the third of the angels that rebelled with Lucifer. They did not have an evil spirit; they were tempted by Lucifer's thoughts to rebel against Father God, and they chose to follow Lucifer. Today, regardless of evil spirits, we still have a personal decision to make. Will we follow

Father God, or will we follow Satan's kingdom through temptation?

In the Millennium, there will be evil spirits, and there will also be human sinners. It is unscriptural to think there will not be any sin in the Millennium. In fact, the Bible says the sinner that dies at 100 is accursed. A child that dies at 100 is accursed.

> *There shall be no more thence an infant of days, nor an old man that hath not filled his days: for the child shall die an hundred years old; but the sinner being an hundred years old shall be accursed.*
> *Isaiah 65:20 KJV*

NATURAL MAN

It is my position that it will be possible to live in the Millennium as a natural man and woman for 1,000 years and never die. After that 1,000 years, they will be judged with the rest of creation — and if they are found faithful, they will live on into eternity. That is natural man. We do not need to worry about it; we will be the redeemed at that point. We will live forever in a glorified body. I am addressing natural people coming out of the Tribulation, who come out of the islands of the sea, and all the nations of the earth which we rule over as Kings and Priests. Those who come out of Egypt, Cuba, all over to the islands of Australia, all over Russia, and every other location around the world — we rule over them. And, the Kingdom of God will be established in the midst of it all. Most churches teach this subject very well. The point is that sinners in the Millennium will have to choose to follow Father God. But what about the New Heavens and New Earth? This time period is only mentioned briefly, but it comes after the Millennial Reign of Christ.

> *Nevertheless we, according to his promise, look for new heavens and a new earth, wherein dwelleth righteousness. 2 Peter 3:13 KJV*

At that point, Satan is gone, and so are all evil spirits. When this matter is settled at the end of the Millennium, there will be no evil spirits left on this planet. Satan, every evil spirit and fallen angel, and everything that followed him will be in the Lake of Fire.

> *And the devil that deceived them was cast into the lake of fire and brimstone, where the beast and the false prophet are, and shall be tormented day and night for ever and ever. Revelation 20:10 KJV*

> *And whosoever was not found written in the book of life was cast into the lake of fire. Revelation 20:15 KJV*

That is what the Bible teaches. All those left are the natural people who were obedient in the Millennium and the saints who rule over them that populate the New Heavens and New Earth. And the

New Jerusalem comes down. A rough conversion of dimensions from the Bible is roughly 1,500 miles wide, 1,500 miles long, and 1,500 miles in depth.

> *Him that overcometh will I make a pillar in the temple of my God, and he shall go no more out: and I will write upon him the name of my God, and the name of the city of my God, which is new Jerusalem, which cometh down out of heaven from my God: and I will write upon him my new name. Revelation 3:12 KJV*

Outside the gates of the city is where the rest of the planet and natural men live. The only way for them to have eternal life is to be able to come through the gates and enter the city to partake of the Tree of Life. Outside the gates are the whoremongers, sorcerers, those who make a lie, and the adulterers.

> *[14]Blessed are they that do his commandments, that they may have right to the tree of life, and may enter in through the gates into the city. [15]For without are dogs, and sorcerers, and whoremongers, and murderers, and idolaters, and whosoever loveth and maketh a lie. Revelation 22:14-15 KJV*

Who will we rule over in the New Heavens and New Earth? Natural men — and some of them are evil. The Bible mentions that sorcerers and liars are outside the city. Even though Satan's kingdom is gone in the New Heavens and New Earth, there is still evil. Creation will still have a battle with evil past Satan and his kingdom, with beings following after evil. We may even find it in ourselves. What if an evil man tempted us, as a King or a Priest, to turn against the living God whom we serve? Could we be tempted? Could we be bribed? Could we be fooled? Could a female of the natural order tempt us to sin? As in the angels who left their proper state of habitation and came down and cohabited with the daughters of men and had the "men of renown" or the "mighty men" of mythology. It is my position that the "sons of God" who fornicated with the daughters of men are the same angels who are reserved in chains in the Book of Jude.

> *There were giants in the earth in those days; and also after that, when the sons of God came in unto the daughters of men, and they bare children to them, the same became mighty men which were of old, men of renown. Genesis 6:4*

> *And the angels which kept not their first estate, but left their own habitation, he hath reserved in everlasting chains under darkness unto the judgment of the great day. Jude 1:6 KJV*

Could we be tempted, children of God, as the angels were to cohabit with the natural men or women in lust? Do we realize that angels lusted? They were not exempt from temptation because they were not humans. We are getting a wonderful chance to practice righteousness in this lifetime. If we are going to bring others out of the "hell of the curse", we need a foundation of truth to stand against the devil. I am making a decision every day to be a son of God. I am not perfect, and I weave as I move forward with God. I am moving forward in my life little by little. As I like to say, "One step backward and two steps forward is still *forward progress.*" Even if we fall, it is time to get back up and keep going. The Bible says the man who puts his hand to the plow and looks back is not fit for the Kingdom of God.

> *And Jesus said unto him, No man, having put his hand to the plough, and looking back, is fit for the kingdom of God. Luke 9:62 KJV*

Remember Lot's wife? She looked back and was not fit for the Kingdom of God. I am going to plow all the way into eternity. Will we listen to lies? Or will we take hold of this reality check, embrace conviction, and established in our hearts where we are headed?

WE MUST CHOOSE

My point is that evil can occur apart from Satan and even evil spirits. This point relates to identity because we must choose to solidify our position before Father God as His child. Otherwise, we will fall into sin because we have not practiced loving Father God and following His ways. I have taught that thoughts come from three dimensions.

How many people are unsure if they listen to themselves, God, or the devil half the time? Well, I have the same problem. I am unsure half the time whether I am in faith or not. I only know if I am in faith when I see the fruit of it. If I knew if I was in faith, I would not need faith, would I? What is faith? Many people in the Word of Faith movement have created a system of works to attain faith. For instance, they might have 14 steps to faith. That is not Biblical; faith is very simple. Hebrews 11:1 sets us straight. This one Scripture defines faith succinctly. It says, "Now faith is the substance of things hoped for, the evidence of things not seen."

> *Now faith is the substance of things hoped for, the evidence of things not seen. Hebrews 11:1 KJV*

Do we have hopes? Then we have faith. What if we lack hope? Then we do not have faith. Lord, increase our faith. There is a saying I have heard regarding faith: "Increase the parameters of the revelation of our hope." I know where I am going in my life. I do not rely on superstition. I do not use divination to understand it. I know it from reading and believing the Word of God. I often find in the Christian Church that they do not know where they have come from, where they are at, or where they are going. They are lost in time and space. I am not lost in time and space. I am not lost in eternity. I know exactly where I am at in my generation in terms of the past, present, and future of this planet. It is time to allow the Word of God to establish our perspective of ourselves and our existence.

NEW HEAVENS AND NEW EARTH

Now, returning to the Book of Revelation, we need to cover the New Heavens and New Earth in chapter 21 verse 7. It says, "He that overcometh shall inherit all things; and I will be his God, and he shall be my son."

He that overcometh shall inherit all things; and I will be his God, and he shall be my son. Revelation 21:7 KJV

That is a great scripture. However, verse 8 serves to caution us to obey God. It is a warning of the consequences to those who rebel against God without turning from sin. It says, "But the fearful, and unbelieving, and the abominable, and murderers, and whoremongers, and sorcerers, and idolaters, and all liars, shall have their part in the lake which burneth with fire and brimstone: which is the second death."

But the fearful, and unbelieving, and the abominable, and murderers, and whoremongers, and sorcerers, and idolaters, and all liars, shall have their part in the lake which burneth with fire and brimstone: which is the second death. Revelation 21:8 KJV

In order to understand our identity, we need to understand where we are going in eternity. In order to understand our future, we need to understand the future of the planet. The New Jerusalem is the centerpiece of the future. Many people view this as metaphor of the Body of Christ that will be fulfilled symbolically in the future. I do not agree. From Scripture, it is a literal city. How do I know it is a literal city? Because it has physical dimensions and it has gates. The city does not need the sun nor the moon to shine in it.

> *And the city had no need of the sun, neither of the moon, to shine in it: for the glory of God did lighten it, and the Lamb is the light thereof. Revelation 21:23 KJV*

By the way, this Scripture does not mean the sun and moon are gone. It just means the brightness of the city and location is that bright. From Scripture, it is a literal location on the planet Earth. Consider this in regard to the planet, the sun, and the moon. Will the planet still be spherical? If that is so, then how could the light of the New Jerusalem illuminate the other side of the planet? I believe the sun and moon are still there for natural people. There will be days and nights, but in the location of the New Jerusalem there will be no day or night because of the brightness thereof. Outside the city, the natural planet will have been restored. This is an aside from my main point, but it is important to address the logic of Scripture and reality. The city will have no need for the sun. However, it does not say the rest of the planet has no need for the sun. It just says the city does not need the sun. The nations of them who are saved shall walk in the light of it. And the kings of the earth shall bring their glory and honor into it. *Into it* means they are coming from outside. *The kings of the earth shall bring their glory into it* means they are coming from the outside and bringing something into it. So, we know the city does not cover the whole earth. It just covers that specific location.

> *And the nations of them which are saved shall walk in the light of it: and the kings of the earth do bring their glory and honour into it. Revelation 21:24 KJV*

I used to have a map covering the Mediterranean, Israel, and Jerusalem. Using it, I pinpointed Jerusalem, took the coordinates from Scripture, and mapped the scale with a thread. I found my coordinates and drew a square. I had it on the wall in my office. It gave me a literal image of what Scripture describes. Revelation 21:25-27 says the gates shall not be shut at all by day, for there shall be no night there. And they shall bring the glory and honor of the nations into it. (That would be from the outside into it.) And it says there shall no wise enter in anything which defileth, neither whatsoever worketh abomination or maketh a lie: but they which are written in the Lamb's Book of Life.

> *25And the gates of it shall not be shut at all by day: for there shall be no night there. 26And they shall bring the glory*

and honour of the nations into it. ²⁷*And there shall in no wise enter into it any thing that defileth, neither whatsoever worketh abomination, or maketh a lie: but they which are written in the Lamb's book of life. Revelation 21:25-27 KJV*

It continues in chapter 22, verse 14: "Blessed are they that do his commandments, that they may have right to the tree of life."

Blessed are they that do his commandments, that they may have right to the tree of life, and may enter in through the gates into the city. Revelation 22:14 KJV

The Tree of Life is in the city. Who entered in through the gates of the city? Natural men. New Jerusalem is our future home. I want to be at the 1,300-mile elevation. I will let the Father have the penthouse. Do we realize how many people this structure will be able to handle? In Revelation 21:16, it measures the city as 12,000 furlongs. Most of us do not use furlongs as a unit of measurement, but it translates to 1,500 miles.

And the city lieth foursquare, and the length is as large as the breadth: and he measured the city with the reed, twelve thousand furlongs. The length and the breadth and the height of it are equal. Revelation 21:16 KJV

If we were to figure each level in 1,500 miles, that is a gigantic structure. It is 1,500 miles long by 1,500 miles wide by 1,500 miles high in the shape of a cube. If we consider the dimensions of a level at one mile high and 1,500 long, wide, and deep as a single part of the city, do we realize how many millions of people the city can handle in terms of the redeemed saints, both Old and New Testament? That is our eternal home. If we believe we are going to heaven to stay forever, the Bible does not teach that. If the Lord returned right now in the First Resurrection, the longest we would be in heaven is seven years. Then we would be right back here in the Millennium. After the Millennium, would be the New Heavens and New Earth. This little jewel, the planet Earth, will be the center headquarters of the universe.

The Lord Jesus will be our spiritual husband. We shall follow Him as Kings and Priests to execute and rule His Kingdom. I believe eventually the universe will be filled with Kings and Priests over planets filled with natural men in the eternal future. We are talking about people continuing to populate planets forever. It sure beats hell. It also sure beats the Lake of Fire. I have decided to stay topside forever, rather than bottomside in the Lake of Fire. That is my hope, that is my faith, that is my joy, and that is my heart to reign with Christ into the eternal future. It is His heart for everyone, too, because it is not just for me. It is for whosoever He beckons who will respond to Him.

It is my position that when natural men die in the New Heavens and New Earth, they will not die a natural death. They will be cast directly into the Lake of Fire. The second death is the Lake of Fire.

> *But the fearful, and unbelieving, and the abominable, and murderers, and whoremongers, and sorcerers, and idolaters, and all liars, shall have their part in the lake which burneth with fire and brimstone: which is the second death. Revelation 21:8 KJV*

The first death is the one we experience in this time period before the Millennial Reign of Christ. The Bible says the smoke of their torment in the Lake of Fire shall vent out of certain parts of the earth forever.

> *And the smoke of their torment ascendeth up for ever and ever: and they have no rest day nor night, who worship the beast and his image, and whosoever receiveth the mark of his name. Revelation 14:11 KJV*

Natural men shall hear the cries of their torment. Unfortunately, there will be those who will still follow evil thoughts apart from devils. In the New Heavens and the New Earth, those outside the city will be known as dogs.

> *14Blessed are they that do his commandments, that they may have right to the tree of life, and may enter in*

through the gates into the city. ¹⁵For
without are dogs, and sorcerers, and
whoremongers, and murderers, and
idolaters, and whosoever loveth and
maketh a lie. Revelation 22:14-15 KJV

That dog is not a "whoof whoof" type of
animal. That word *dog* is a pretty strong term that
means spiritually corrupt. As a matter of fact, the
word *heathen* means *dog*. It means being spiritually
separated from the living God and following the
living principle of evil. "For without are dogs, and
sorcerers, and whoremongers, and murderers, and
idolaters, and whosoever loveth and maketh a lie."
Verse 17 is one of my favorite scriptures in the Bible.
It says, "And the Spirit and the bride say, Come. Let
him that heareth say, Come. And let him that is
athirst come. And whosoever will, let him take the
water of life freely."

And the Spirit and the bride say, Come.
And let him that heareth say, Come. And
let him that is athirst come. And
whosoever will, let him take the water of
life freely. Revelation 22:17 KJV

KNOW OUR ENEMY

And the *capitalized* Spirit and the Bride say,
"Come." We, as the Body of Christ, are the Bride. I
want to take people, in the spirit of their hearts, into
the future at this level. I do not want to wait until the
future. I want everyone to get this picture in the

present. I want the principalities and the powers to be defeated right now. I want God's greater grace to come into our lives, not just His sustaining grace. I intend to give the truth, so the truth will make us free. I want everyone to know their enemy. I want everyone to understand their thoughts. I want everyone to be able to defeat everything in their lives that does not match the mind of the living God who created them. And if I may bring people to that place of application in the Lord, the devil will be defeated — and diseases, insanities, and problems will begin to fall off people's bodies.

Many who have spent time around this ministry have experienced this revelation, and their lives have been altered forever. Now, this statement is not meant to build up this ministry. It is not meant to build me up. It is meant to build Him up because Christ is the head of the Church, and I am just a small part of the bigger picture. We do not begin with the prophetic future. Without this complete teaching, we cannot have the discerning of spirits. We will not even know what or who they are. We have become so one with spirits, we believe they are us. We have all these feelings and thoughts that come into our heads.

Someone may say that is just the way they are. Is listening to temptation having the mind of Christ? Does Christ have a spirit of fear? Does Christ have self-hatred? Does Christ have jealousy? Does He have any of the things that are wrong with humanity? No. Do we believe the Lord loves being married to a diseased wife? Do we believe that is the conversation between Satan and the Lord? Do we believe the Lord is in heaven saying, "Look at my diseased Church, I will heal her when she gets to heaven?" And then Satan would say, "Yes, bless God, I will kill them while they are here." Do we believe that is the doctrine of our God? I cannot find that in Scripture anywhere, and I will not teach it. I will state this: we have opened the door to the devil in our generations from Adam. We have opened the door to the devil in our generations and personal lives. It is time to get a reality check. What will we choose? Choose this day what to have: life or death, blessings or cursings.

> *I call heaven and earth to record this day against you, that I have set before you life and death, blessing and cursing: therefore choose life, that both thou and thy seed may live: Deuteronomy 30:19 KJV*

CHAPTER 11: The Nature of God

HATRED FOR EVIL

Remember Romans 1:21-22? It says, "They glorified him not as God, neither were thankful; but became vain in their imaginations, and their foolish heart was darkened. Professing themselves to be wise, they became fools."

> *²¹Because that, when they knew God, they glorified him not as God, neither were thankful; but became vain in their imaginations, and their foolish heart was darkened. ²²Professing themselves to be wise, they became fools, Romans 1:21-22 KJV*

The Church professes itself to be wise while it is a foolish Bride. Even if we say we know what God does, it not mean that we are known of God. Jesus said in that day, when they will stand before Him, they will say they have cast out devils in His name, healed the sick in His name, and prophesied in His name. But He will say, "I never knew you: depart from Me, ye that work iniquity."

> *²²Many will say to me in that day, Lord, Lord, have we not prophesied in thy name? and in thy name have cast out devils? and in thy name done many*

wonderful works? *²³And then will I profess unto them, I never knew you: depart from me, ye that work iniquity. Matthew 7:22-23 KJV*

Why would the Lord honor somebody who He does not know? Much of the Church is focused on its own ideas that have little understanding from the Word of God. They do not know Him. As Scripture states, "Professing themselves to be wise, they became fools, And changed the glory of the uncorruptible God into an image made like to corruptible man, and to birds, and fourfooted beasts, and creeping things. Wherefore God also gave them up to uncleanness through the lusts of their own hearts, to dishonor their own bodies between themselves: Who changed the truth of God into a lie."

²² Professing themselves to be wise, they became fools, ²³And changed the glory of the uncorruptible God into an image made like to corruptible man, and to birds, and fourfooted beasts, and creeping things. ²⁴Wherefore God also gave them up to uncleanness through the lusts of their own hearts, to dishonour their own bodies between themselves: ²⁵Who changed the truth of God into a lie, and worshipped and served the creature more than the Creator, who is blessed for ever. Amen. Romans 1:22-25 KJV

They changed the truth into a lie. Did they know the truth? Yes. Did they change the truth? Yes. If someone invalidates the Word of God through false doctrine, it may become the law of their hearts. If we believe them, it will become the word of Satan for our lives. Regardless of what Scriptures we know, if we refuse to follow them, we will follow after sin. Paul said that when he did evil, he consented unto the law of God that the law of Satan was good.

If then I do that which I would not, I consent unto the law that it is good.
Romans 7:16 KJV

When we know the truth and do not do it, we are deceived. We are establishing Satan as the ruler of this planet all over again. We are also crucifying Christ all over again because we refuse to turn away from sin. Instead, we have chosen to follow sin over repentance.

If they shall fall away, to renew them again unto repentance; seeing they crucify to themselves the Son of God afresh, and put him to an open shame.
Hebrews 6:6 KJV

Someone may say, "Well, I do not commit any major sins." Really? Where are the degrees of sin in the Bible? I did not read this; if we offend in one point of the law, we are guilty of all.

For whosoever shall keep the whole
law, and yet offend in one point, he is
guilty of all. James 2:10 KJV

There are no degrees of sin. It is as evil to have
strife between us and another person as it is to
murder someone with a gun. It is equally evil to have
strife, envy, and jealousy amongst ourselves as any
other sin. Let us get this straight. Let us not socialize
sin and psychologize unrighteousness. Let us not
make sin socially acceptable. Let us have, as the Bible
tells us, hatred for evil.

Ye that love the LORD, hate evil: he
preserveth the souls of his saints; he
delivereth them out of the hand of the
wicked. Psalm 97:10 KJV

DISCERNING OF SPIRITS

Can I teach this without it producing legalism?
May I teach this without putting people in a place
where they feel condemned? I hope so because that is
not my heart, nor is it God's heart. It is not loving for
me to ignore truth so as not to offend anyone. I am
teaching discernment. Beginning in Romans 1:25, it
says, "Who changed the truth of God into a lie, and
worshipped and served the creature more than the
Creator, who is blessed for ever. Amen. For this cause
God gave them up unto vile affections: for even their
women did change the natural use into that which is
against nature: And likewise also the men, leaving the
natural use of the woman, burned in their lust one

toward another; men with men working that which is unseemly, and receiving in themselves that recompense of their error which was meet. And even as they did not like to retain God in their knowledge, God gave them over to a reprobate mind."

²⁵Who changed the truth of God into a lie, and worshipped and served the creature more than the Creator, who is blessed for ever. Amen. ²⁶For this cause God gave them up unto vile affections: for even their women did change the natural use into that which is against nature: ²⁷And likewise also the men, leaving the natural use of the woman, burned in their lust one toward another; men with men working that which is unseemly, and receiving in themselves that recompence of their error which was meet. ²⁸And even as they did not like to retain God in their knowledge, God gave them over to a reprobate mind, to do those things which are not convenient; Romans 1:25-28 KJV

Let me say this: if we continue to believe a lie of Satan and his "gospel", God will withdraw and release us to whatever gospel we want. If we would rather believe a lie, then God will give us over to a greater delusion to believe a greater lie so that the greater destruction will be ours. If we want to follow the word of Satan, then we make him our "father", and he will "bless" us. But his blessing to us is the curse. When we have had enough of the curse of following Satan, which is his blessing, maybe we will come back to God. If we repent to Him, we will receive true blessings, which is freedom from the curse. God will let us have what we want. If we do not want to forgive our neighbor, He will not stop us. If someone wants to have envy and jealousy, go right ahead. If someone wants to have evil in their heart, go right ahead. If someone wants to hate themselves, go right ahead. If someone wants to hate their brother, go right ahead. If someone wants to hate God, go right ahead. He has created us to be free-will agents, and we can make our own choices. We can do what we want. "According to your faith be it unto you."

> *Then touched he their eyes, saying,*
> *According to your faith be it unto you.*
> *Matthew 9:29 KJV*

We quote that Scripture from the standpoint of receiving, do we not? What if we reverse it and address sin? When we disobey, can it be said: according to our faith in Satan, so be it unto us? It is according to our faith. If we sow unto darkness, we shall reap darkness. If we sow unto light, we shall reap light. Like begets like. If we sow in darkness, we shall reap darkness. If we sow in love, we shall reap love. If we sow in bitterness, we shall reap bitterness. If we sow in unforgiveness, we shall reap unforgiveness. If we sow in deception, we shall reap deception. If we sow in hatred, we shall reap hatred. "Whatsoever a man soweth, that shall he also reap."

Be not deceived; God is not mocked: for whatsoever a man soweth, that shall he also reap. Galatians 6:7 KJV

Romans 1:29 says, "Being filled with all unrighteousness, fornication, wickedness, covetousness, maliciousness; full of envy, murder, debate, deceit, malignity; whisperers, Backbiters, haters of God, despiteful, proud, boasters, inventers of evil things, disobedient to parents, Without understanding, covenantbreakers, without natural affection, implacable, unmerciful: Who knowing the judgment of God, that they which commit such things are worthy of death, not only do the same, but have pleasure in them that do them."

²⁹Being filled with all unrighteousness, fornication, wickedness, covetousness, maliciousness; full of envy, murder, debate, deceit, malignity; whisperers, ³⁰Backbiters, haters of God, despiteful, proud, boasters, inventors of evil things, disobedient to parents, ³¹Without understanding, covenantbreakers, without natural affection, implacable, unmerciful: ³²Who knowing the judgment of God, that they which commit such things are worthy of death, not only do the same, but have pleasure in them that do them. Romans 1:29-32 KJV

Discernment involves having the mind of Christ. The issues stated in Romans 1 are not the mind of Christ. Has any of that stuff been in our lives at some point? Maybe it still is. That is what we are after – those sins are the leaven and the spots and blemishes. These also open the door to the curse.

SIN IS GUILTY

As I listed earlier, all manner of diseases listed in Deuteronomy 28 are the curse. All manner of diseases are the result of disobedience to God's Word. All kinds of diseases are disobedience to God's Word. However, what does disobedience to God's Word mean? It has to do with our relationships. When we looked at Romans 1, does it have to do with contact with someone else? Debate, contention, strife – it is conflict at some level. Do not many of them relate to conflicts in relationships?

Romans said the knowledge of sin came through the giving of the law.

Therefore by the deeds of the law there shall no flesh be justified in his sight: for by the law is the knowledge of sin.
Romans 3:20 KJV

God wants us to know what is right and wrong, not because He wants to oppress us with goodness. No, He wants to show us what is right. We are thinking people; do we want someone to tell us what is right? That is, anyone except God. There are many people who go to everyone but God to let them know what is right. What I find in Scripture is the best for mankind. The nature of God is the best that mankind could ever be. What is wrong with being the best that mankind could ever be? What is wrong with loving each other? What is wrong with forgiving each other? Why do we have to be in strife? Do we know why people go into strife? Because somebody is trying to establish their own kingdom, not God's kingdom. Because God came as a servant and people in strife do not want to serve anybody. They want to serve themselves, and they want to exalted. The Bible says we are to prefer other people over ourselves.

> *Let nothing be done through strife or vainglory; but in lowliness of mind let each esteem other better than themselves. Philippians 2:3 KJV*

We are to serve each other. We are the gifts of the living God to natural man forever. So the question is, are we going to build up mankind, or are we going to pull them down? There are a lot of people who are going to have to stand before the Lord one day and give an account for how they pulled down others. I do not want to be in their shoes. The Bible says if we judge ourselves, God will not have to judge us.

> *For if we would judge ourselves, we should not be judged. 1 Corinthians 11:31 KJV*

That is what the Word says, so I am busy judging myself. However, because I am judging myself does not mean I am living in condemnation. Is it possible to judge ourselves, still have sin, and not be in condemnation? Is it possible to have a healthy judgment? Is it possible to scrutinize ourselves spiritually, look at something evil in ourselves, and not feel bad about ourselves? Well, it should be.

If we have become one with sin, we will feel bad about ourselves. Condemnation binds us to the sin. Conviction separates us from sin. There is a different spirit behind one than the spirit behind the other. The devil is behind one; God is behind the other. The devil is there to condemn us when we fall, and God is there to convict us. Isn't it amazing how the devil will tempt us — and then when we have fallen, he will condemn us? Do we know who the guiltiest being on the planet is? It is the devil and his kingdom. It is the craziest thing. His kingdom convinces us to sin, and then when we are done, he blames us for the action he instigated. However, Paul turned the coin on him. My paraphrase is that he said, "It was not me who did that sin anyway. It was that sin who did it through me, so *it* is guilty."

> [19]*For the good that I would I do not: but the evil which I would not, that I do.* [20]*Now if I do that I would not, it is no more I that do it, but sin that dwelleth in me.* [21]*I find then a law, that, when I would do good, evil is present with me.* **Romans 7:19-21 KJV**

I want everyone to repeat this out loud for their freedom. I would like everyone to say: "For every sin that is in my life, if you are a being — you are the guilty one. And if I am the cause of it, I am the guilty one. But God has made a provision for me. He has made no provision for them because they are judged forever. I am under grace and under mercy and have a lifetime to work out my salvation. I have a lifetime to defeat the curse that is in the earth. Father God, open my heart today. Bring conviction to my heart. As for condemnation, shut up! Father God, do not stop talking to me. Holy Spirit, You were given to me to lead me into all truth. I do not intend to believe a lie. It is detrimental to my health. I want to believe truth. Truth feels good. To know the truth will make me free. Father, help me develop a perfect hatred for evil. Cleanse me, purge me, make me a vessel of honor, and when I fall or I fail—and I probably will—remind me to rise again. The Word says in Proverbs 24:16 that the righteous fall or fail seven times and rise up again. Jesus told Peter in Luke 22:31 that Satan desired to sift him like wheat. That was not a negative confession. That was a statement of spiritual existence because the Lord told Peter that after he had recovered himself, he should strengthen the brethren. When I have recovered myself, I am going to strengthen the brethren. I may fall, and that is not a negative confession. That is a statement of my spiritual condition. And in my honesty before You, Father God, You will meet me and help me to rise again seven times. Amen."

WORSHIPING THE CREATURE

Remember that Hebrews 4:13 says, "Neither is there any creature that is not made manifest in his sight: but all things are naked and opened unto the eyes of him with whom we have to do."

Neither is there any creature that is not manifest in his sight: but all things are naked and opened unto the eyes of him with whom we have to do. Hebrews 4:13 KJV

When we go back to Romans 1:25, it says, "Who changed the truth of God into a lie, and worshipped and served the creature more than the Creator."

Who changed the truth of God into a lie, and worshipped and served the creature more than the Creator, who is blessed for ever. Amen. Romans 1:25 KJV

Who is the creature in this verse? It is an evil spirit from Satan and his kingdom. It is the body of sin. When we follow after unforgiveness, we serve the creature of unforgiveness, and we change the forgiveness of the living God into a lie by disobeying the instruction of the Bible. The word *creature* is the same Greek word in both the Romans and Hebrews Scriptures stated above. It is Greek 2937 in the Strong's Concordance. It is from Greek 2936 at the root. This root word refers to manufacturing or fabricating, otherwise defined as "to make." The word 2937 means original formation. How does this apply to our understanding of this subject? The creature in Romans 1:25 can be any type of created being. At its core, it would be something that has been fabricated or created.

Therefore, if we are worshiping the creature rather than the Creator, how could the term *creature* be interpreted correctly? Could that include worshiping each other? Yes, it could include worshiping and idolizing other humans. It could also include worshiping mythological gods and goddesses. However, behind these gods and goddesses, which are fictional creatures, are the very real forces that produce ungodly fruit in our lives. And just as we separate ourselves and other people from sin, we can also see the spirits behind these ideologies and thought processes. There are spirits behind false gods. In the context of this Scripture in Romans, the term *creature* is mentioned in conjunction with sin. With that understood, let us bring this Scripture into context. This Scripture describes worshiping the creature rather than the Creator, which is a specific *work of the flesh.*

WORKS OF THE FLESH

In Galatians 5:19, I want to focus on the first 4-5 words. Let us read this carefully: "Now the works of the flesh are manifest."

Now the works of the flesh are manifest, which are these; Adultery, fornication, uncleanness, lasciviousness, Galatians 5:19 KJV

The works of the flesh are Satan's nature manifested through us. They come from the invisible creatures manifesting their natures through us, which would, in turn, make us also a sinful being in the area of our lives where we yield to their temptation. Now, this statement is predicated upon our will and decision. We may have every temptation of an evil spirit and not yield to sin. It is *sin* to us when we act out their thoughts and allow those invisible beings to use us as a medium of expression for themselves. When we act out their nature, it becomes our sin.

In my previous teaching on the 7 Steps to Sin, I define the process of yielding to temptation and going into sin. Without reteaching the subject, James 1:14-15 describes the process of being tempted. It involves a progressive yielding to feelings and thoughts from Satan's kingdom. It begins with being drawn away of our own lusts, being enticed, then lust is conceived in our hearts, and then it brings forth sin. Before the final part, we have not yet committed sin. Many people have been tempted, and they think they have sinned. For instance, many people are given awful thoughts as temptation, and they believe they have sinned because they have a terrible idea in their minds. Unless we act upon the thoughts and fulfill them in our lives, it is just temptation.

> *14But every man is tempted, when he is drawn away of his own lust, and enticed. 15Then when lust hath conceived, it bringeth forth sin: and sin,*

when it is finished, bringeth forth death.
James 1:14-15 KJV

Temptation is not sin. How do I know that? Because the Bible says Jesus was tempted in all points, such as we are, yet without sin. So I know temptation is not sin; otherwise, Jesus would not be sinless because He was also tempted.

For we have not an high priest which
cannot be touched with the feeling of
our infirmities; but was in all points
tempted like as we are, yet without sin.
Hebrews 4:15 KJV

What if a spirit of lust came to tempt us? What if we did not have a spirit of lust, but one came to tempt us? Do we know how lust comes? It comes with very emotional pictures and "video playback" in our minds with every feeling and every rush we can imagine. It would feel just as real as if we really had the problem. Now, what are we going to do with it? We either become one with it and act it out, or we recognize it as the creature working to gain access to our lives, resist it, get rid of it, and turn away. That is resisting temptation. What is temptation? Many people do not understand the definition of temptation. Temptation could be anything that changes the Word of God into a lie. Anything that defies the instruction of the Word of God is a form of temptation. It could be any sinful conduct in our lives. It could be something as simple as bitterness, envy, jealousy, or fear.

I want to make it abundantly clear that behind the scenes of our world and lives, there is an evil kingdom — and that kingdom wants us. That same kingdom needs us. It is the body of sin, and it cannot manifest on the earth unless it has a human being; no more than the Body of Christ can manifest in the earth unless there is a human being involved with God as a work of the Holy Spirit. We are either part of the Body of Christ or we are part of the body sin by decision. We choose every day as we follow after sin. We all have sin. In Revelation 19, the Bride of Christ is making herself ready by getting the spots and the blemishes out of her life.

> *7Let us be glad and rejoice, and give honour to him: for the marriage of the Lamb is come, and his wife hath made herself ready. 8And to her was granted that she should be arrayed in fine linen, clean and white: for the fine linen is the righteousness of saints. Revelation 19:7-8 KJV*

Do we take our clothes to the dry cleaners when they have spots and blemishes? Do we wash our clothes when they are dirty? Why not do the same thing with ourselves spiritually? If we take time and effort for our clothes, why should we not take time for our spirits and souls? We should take as much time to address the invisible as we do with the visible.

WE OUGHT TO BE TEACHERS

As we conclude, it is time to tie together some subjects. In order to tie these subjects to our identity, we need to go to Romans 7, then go back to Romans 6, and return to Romans 1. Romans 7 brings us back into focus because of what Paul said about himself and his spiritual battles. If Paul had spiritual battles as an apostle, who else has spiritual battles? We do. I believe that sometimes we are afraid to face the parts of us that are not really us. Condemnation makes us one with the sin. Conviction separates us from the sin. This is becoming a powerful axiom of truth. In other words, condemnation binds us to and makes us one with the sin. And what is sin? Sin is a being, and the state of being of the *being of sin* tempts us. When we agree with it, it manifests through us, and performs actions that contradict the nature of God. If God's nature is forgiveness, which it is, and I do not forgive my brother, then I am into sin.

What is another facet of sin? It is anything that falls short of the glory of God. What is the glory of God? The glory of God is the nature of God. What does it mean if we are being changed from glory to glory into His image? Well, if we are being changed from glory to glory into His image, then there was something within us or part of us that was not according to His image; otherwise, we would not need to change.

But we all, with open face beholding as in a glass the glory of the Lord, are changed into the same image from glory

*to glory, even as by the Spirit of the
Lord. 2 Corinthians 3:18 KJV*

Does my conclusion seem logical? Sometimes we become so busy chasing truth we do not take time to sit with it and make it part of us. At some point, we become so busy filling ourselves with knowledge that it becomes vanity to us because we do not have the opportunity to apply it and make it a practical part of our lives. How much truth have we been taught that we have forgotten? In other words, how much truth do we know in our heads that we are not walking in? This is just an honest observation I have made. So, how does truth become part of our lives? Hebrews 5:13-14 tells us how. It comes by day-to-day, practical application with other humans to discern both good and evil.

> [13]*For every one that useth milk is
> unskilful in the word of righteousness:
> for he is a babe.* [14]*But strong meat
> belongeth to them that are of full age,
> even those who by reason of use have
> their senses exercised to discern both
> good and evil. Hebrews 5:13-14 KJV*

To understand these verses, we need to go back further. In Hebrews 5, there is a powerful insight beginning in verse 11. It says, "Of whom we have many things to say, and hard to be uttered, seeing ye are dull of hearing."

*Of whom we have many things to say,
and hard to be uttered, seeing ye are dull
of hearing. Hebrews 5:11 KJV*

Well, that is kind of a blunt statement. In verse 12, it says, "For when for the time ye ought to be teachers, ye have need that one teach you again."

*For when for the time ye ought to be
teachers, ye have need that one teach
you again which be the first principles
of the oracles of God; and are become
such as have need of milk, and not of
strong meat. Hebrews 5:12 KJV*

Many of us have heard so much truth that we ought to be teachers. All of us have enough truth in us to win the whole world to Christ. All we need is John 3:16.

*For God so loved the world, that he
gave his only begotten Son, that
whosoever believeth in him should not
perish, but have everlasting life. John
3:16 KJV*

That is all we need. There is more to truth than just John 3:16. John 3:16 is a statement of God's love, His position for us, and our position in Him through Christ. However, for many of us, there is enough information from the Bible within us that we ought to be able to teach others.

I do not spend time listening to tapes or books of others. I have done that in my earlier journey as a believer. I have spent years learning. My library is filled with tapes and books from a variety of Christian individuals covering what they have said about many subjects. I have done my homework about what men have said about God and religions and societies and civilizations, and I have spent time in my personal study. Today the only study I really do is the Word of God. I do not believe I have used anything but the Word in 10 years. I read no other books. I do not have time. By the time I have read a book, I have usually already found it in the Word of God. I am interested in other people's revelations, but I will honestly say the most dangerous place in the world today is a Christian bookstore. I do not bother going into them. They are dangerous to my spiritual health because there are many books on a subject, and each contradicts the other. A Christian bookstore is not the purveyor of truth anymore. It is a purveyor of error, from translations to everybody's idioms and theology, with publishers trying to make money by coming up with whatever. I do not bother with it. It is a dangerous place to go, and all it is doing is sowing confusion within the sheep, otherwise known as Christians. Just because it has the word "Christian" attached to it and it touches on the subject of God, we may think it is holy. I think a comic strip probably has more truth in it than most Christian bookstores.

I do not want to be overly negative because there is also good stuff in those same Christian bookstores, but we have to pick through it. We must pick through it and discern. If we spent more time reading our Bibles and letting the Holy Spirit teach us than listening to tapes, watching videos, and reading books, we might learn something. If we have a good, solid King James Bible and a Strong's Concordance and begin to read Scripture in context and look up the words we do not understand in the Concordance, it is amazing what God can teach us. The small amount of time most Christians spend in Bible study today is embarrassing to discuss. If we spent as much time reading our Bibles as we do watching television shows, we would be in better spiritual shape.

Hebrews 5:12 says, "For when for the time ye ought to be teachers, ye have need that one teach you again which be the first principles of the oracles of God."

> *For when for the time ye ought to be teachers, ye have need that one teach you again which be the first principles of the oracles of God; and are become such as have need of milk, and not of strong meat. Hebrews 5:12 KJV*

BY REASON OF USE

I want to focus on the term *first principles*. I believe the Church needs to go back to basics again. The Church needs to come back to basic, foundational truth. I believe we have left it behind. We cannot get caught up in all the arguments found in our average Christian bookstore. With that said, I want to refocus on my main point. I read Scripture to bring this subject into context. "But strong meat belongeth to them that are of full age, even those who by reason of use have their senses exercised to discern both good and evil."

> *But strong meat belongeth to them that are of full age, even those who by reason of use have their senses exercised to discern both good and evil. Hebrews 5:14 KJV*

Consider the words *reason of use*. This is where I meant to focus our attention. I want to ensure that at this point in this teaching on *Our Identity*, I can give a practical takeaway for application in our lives. We need principles to apply to our lives every day. Do we believe we only need to discern our lives just on Sundays from 10:00 am until 1:00 pm when we are in a church service? Or do we need to be able to discern 24 hours a day, seven days a week? "But strong meat belongeth to them that are of full age, even those who by reason of use have their senses exercised to discern both good and evil."

The term *senses* in Hebrews 5:14 is a Greek word talking about the five physical senses, but it also corresponds to the entire dimension of our existence. That includes everything that we are in spirit, soul, and body. We must be awake. Our eyes must be open, not in fear or suspicion, but we must be awake to what is operating in the world today. How many of us drive down the road going to town with our eyes shut? We will not get too far, will we? Additionally, how many of us speed up and keep on going when we see a stop sign? I used to see the word *stop* as the acronym S.T.O.P. or "slowly travel on, please." It is also known as a California-style "rolling stop." Are we changing the Word of God or bending it to fit our needs? We need to heed God's warnings rather than ignore them. If it says stop, we need to stop moving. God created us to be very intelligent, spiritual, and wide-awake individuals. I love my brain. I would be in a difficult place without it. It does not always work the way I want it to, but that is because I have not exercised it in certain needed areas. Now, I know that when we pray in the Spirit, our spirit prays unto God. According to Jude, when we pray in the Holy Ghost, we also build up ourselves in the most holy faith.

But ye, beloved, building up yourselves on your most holy faith, praying in the Holy Ghost, Jude 1:20 KJV

I have been teaching about the human spirit, but it important to understand how this connects to the other parts of our creation. Our faculties and ability to think are our connection with the physical world and one another. It is amazing to see how many diseases that are coming upon man involve the breakdown of thought—this includes Parkinson's, Alzheimer's, and many other diseases that are creating plaque on nerve synapses. My personal conclusion is that they are creating an accumulation of white corpuscles on nerve synapses.

As a result of this accumulation, there are many breakups in neurological processes that interrupt our ability to think properly and process thought. These diseases are a part of the curse of sin. Much of what we have discovered in ministering and dealing with these types of neurological diseases is rooted in two areas—one is occultic involvement, such as false religions and New Age practices, and the other is in self-hatred and guilt. As a result of our involvement with these sins, they allow the enemy to come and afflict us at that level.

THE WORD IN OUR HEARTS

In order to change the way I think, I have learned Scripture. I do not like memorization. It is a lot of work. I did not like memorization at all when I had to do it in school. However, as a believer, I have learned to associate with concepts of the Word. These concepts and keywords come to me. I have to look up words in the Concordance to investigate Scriptures. As a minister or as an individual believer—whether I am dealing with someone in ministry or addressing an issue in my own life—when I am moved on by the Holy Spirit, He brings back to my remembrance keywords of a concept. How many of us operate that way? We may not remember an entire verse; we may not even remember a specific book of the Bible.

Oftentimes, we cannot remember exactly where to find a specific verse or concept that is coming to our hearts. However, how many times in the situations of life has a keyword about a subject popped up in our mind? From the keyword, we remembered the rest of the words of Scripture. And if we were unsure, we could take that keyword and go to the internet or a Strong's Concordance and look it up and find the Scripture. I believe that is one of the main ways God speaks to us. I do not believe God intended that we memorize Genesis to Revelation, although I do believe that we should tuck away a large portion of it in our hearts. I believe many of us have a large portion of the Word of God tucked away in our hearts. By tucked away in our hearts, I mean that we have read and considered what Father God said in the Word of God. We may not have memorized it, but we have taken to heart and desired to follow Scripture as we have read it. We may not remember exactly where to find it, and that is why we have resources such as concordances to track down Scriptures.

Many times in ministering, keywords have come to me about subjects so that I could flash the Sword of the Spirit and establish the Kingdom of God and defeat the enemy so a person may be free. Jesus defeated Satan with the Word of God. When he was tempted by Satan in Matthew 4, He would say, "For it is written." And when we say, "For it is written," that establishes the Word in our lives. In fact, the Bible says that God exalts His Word even above His name.

I will worship toward thy holy temple,
and praise thy name for thy
lovingkindness and for thy truth: for

thou hast magnified thy word above all
thy name. Psalm 138:2 KJV

So when we can come in the name of Jesus, who is He? He is God the Word. So, which is greater—His name or His words? Now, I said "who He is" because He is the Lord. He said that we could do all things in His name. But how does that work? The Holy Spirit will only honor the name of Jesus to the degree we honor the Word of God in our lives. I see many people trying to use the name of Jesus as a mantra, mechanism, or modality to move the hand of God. God is not moved by the fact that we use His name. He is moved by the fact that we are obedient to His Word.

CHILDREN OF OBEDIENCE

As we conclude, remember 2 Corinthians 10:5-6? It instructs us to hold every thought in captivity, casting down every imagination and everything that would exalt itself against the knowledge of God.

⁵Casting down imaginations, and every
high thing that exalteth itself against
the knowledge of God, and bringing into
captivity every thought to the obedience
of Christ; ⁶And having in a readiness to
revenge all disobedience, when your
obedience is fulfilled. 2 Corinthians
10:5-6 KJV

The knowledge of God is the Word of God. Then it says, "And having in a readiness to revenge all disobedience, when your obedience is fulfilled." Remember what the Prophet Samuel told King Saul? Obedience is better than sacrifice.

And Samuel said, Hath the LORD as great delight in burnt offerings and sacrifices, as in obeying the voice of the LORD? Behold, to obey is better than sacrifice, and to hearken than the fat of rams. 1 Samuel 15:22 KJV

Obedience to what? The Word of God. If God says in His Word to forgive our neighbor, what are we going to do? Forgive our neighbor. If God says to love our neighbor as ourselves, what are we going to do? Love our neighbor as ourselves. If the Bible says we should love the Lord our God with all of our heart, all of our soul, all of our might, and love our neighbor as ourselves, what are we going to do? If the Bible says to hold every thought in captivity that exalts itself against the knowledge of God, what are we going to do? If the Word of God says, "Blessed are the merciful: for they shall obtain mercy," what are we going to do?

One of the first principles of God I learned years ago is that if I wanted mercy, I had to give it. I learned that in Matthew 5 and I never forgot it. It was there in black and white—if I wanted to receive mercy, what was I supposed to give? Mercy.

Blessed are the merciful: for they shall obtain mercy. Matthew 5:7 KJV

The more mercy I give, the more mercy I receive in return. Is that not wonderful? This is a spiritual principle — an axiom of truth. God watches over His Word to perform it. The Church today is seeing the promises, and they are asking God to watch over His word to perform it, but they do not want to be obedient. They want the conclusion of the promise, but they do not want the predicated obedience that produces it.

As I have laid out throughout this book, God is not asking for perfection. Will we fail? Of course. But He has given us a place of repentance and restoration. He does not just want us to desire His hand in healing, but He also desires to share His nature with us by sanctification. Our identity is tied to Father God and the Word of God. We have been created to be children of God. He does not just want to share some of the benefits with us. He wants to share His heart and eternity with us.

A PRAYER

I want to conclude with a prayer. Father God, for this purpose was the Son of God manifested, that He might destroy the works of the devil. According to Acts 10:38, You anointed Jesus Christ of Nazareth with power and the Holy Ghost, and He went about doing good and healing all who were oppressed of the devil.

Father, sanctify our hearts and increase our faith. Let us start to see our true identity. Let us begin to see what God created from the foundation of the world that we have been ripped off in our lives — either through rejection by others and rejecting others, giving back the same thing, and taking on the victim role because of being victimized by others. Let us be confronted with Your marvelous light of truth. Let us be able to separate ourselves from condemnation and enter into conviction. Let us, of a truth, understand what Paul taught in Romans 7 that what was within was not even him. Let us be able to let light confront darkness, which is so powerful. Let light come together with darkness because the light will dispel the darkness. Let us not run from darkness, but toward it with the glorious light of the Gospel of Jesus Christ. Let us come before that evil kingdom and let us have discernment.

Father, if I could pray a perfect prayer, it would be to ask You to give these people discernment of spirits. It is one of the nine gifts of the Holy Spirit in 1 Corinthians 12. Let us be able to discern both good and evil. Let us not be afraid of evil because that would be ungodly. Why should we be afraid of evil? The Bible has said very clearly that good defeats evil. We are not to defeat evil with evil, but we are to defeat evil with good. Because good always defeats evil, and evil never defeats good. And even though it seems like evil is on the rise and evil is all around, Father God, You are a great God, and where sin abounds, grace much more abounds.

Do we sin that grace might more abound? God forbid. Should we be slaves unto sin, or should we be slaves unto righteousness? God, let us have a paradigm shift in our thinking and let us be open to being slaves to righteousness. If we have been slaves to sin and not cared, why should becoming a slave to righteousness be something we push back against? If there is an anti-Christ spirit of lawlessness and rebellion pushing back against righteousness, please remove it.

Father, give us a heart to let You be our Master. Take away the anti-Christ mentality of rebellion that would not want us to submit to the living God. Take away the evil heart and the hardness of heart of rebellion, pride, witchcraft, and stubbornness, and let our hearts be open to You. We have been created to the glory of Your praise, Father, and Your glory is Your nature manifested in us. Change us so that all men may see that we are of God because of the love we have one for another first. And because our nature matches Your nature, that they may see the good work You have done in us through the Lord Jesus Christ as the work of the Holy Spirit. We want them to glorify You in heaven because they see the good works You have done in our lives. Father, let us want to be like You.

Lord Jesus, give us the desire to be like You. Let us understand that true spirituality is having Your nature. Let us understand that true spirituality is our hearts conforming to You and how You think. God, change our natures. Let us develop a perfect hatred for those aspects of our nature that did not come from You but came from the devil and his kingdom. God, give us a soft heart. Give us a repentant heart. Give us a humble heart. Give us a contrite heart. Give us a heart of faith. Deliver us from an evil heart of unbelief, and open our eyes to the tragedy of mankind. Let us see from the Word of God the tragedy of men's hearts that have been ingrained with the principles and the doctrines of Satan and his kingdom. Let us see how they are the opposite of the Kingdom of our glorious God in heaven.

Father, change us. Father, give us a perfect hatred for evil. Father, sanctify our hearts. Father, change us from glory to glory. Father, we have been created in Your image. Let Your heart be recreated within us as a work of the Holy Spirit. Let us understand Your nature. Let us understand everything that is not Your nature. Let the integrity of our hearts be developed with You and one another. And if we bump into those around us who are unrenewed, those who are held captive, and are slaves to sin, let us have compassion for them. When You came from heaven, Lord, You saw us in our evil, and You had compassion for us. You were able to separate us from evil. And if You were able to separate us from evil and love us, let us be able to separate others from their evil that we may love them. Let us not repay evil for evil. And when those unrenewed ones trample on our spiritual toes and injure us, let us have eyes to see and ears to hear — to recognize that they are blinded to reality. Father, give us soft hearts of compassion for those around us.

Let us be gifts one to another that the Scriptures of Galatians 6:1-2 can be fulfilled: that if a brother be overtaken in a fault, those of you who consider yourselves spiritual, restore such a one in a spirit of meekness and consider yourself also lest you be tempted in like manner and fall away. Bear one another's burdens and, thereby, fulfill the law of Christ.

In the Word, You said we are not to strive over vain disputations of the truth because they lend themselves to more ungodliness. Let us be people who love each other. Father, as we finish this teaching about our identity, challenge us about our identity. And let us not be afraid of things we see in our identity that are not of You. Let us not be condemned, and let us not go into torment, but let us come to a place of conviction. Let us remember what we have been taught by the Spirit of God that condemnation binds us to sin, but conviction separates us from it. Father, deliver us, be with us, guide us by Your Holy Spirit, uphold us with Your free Spirit, and lead us into all truth for Thy name's sake. Amen.

What Be In Health® Offers

Now that you've read *Our Identity*, you may be interested in these other resources that Be in Health has to offer.

FOR MY LIFE®

For My Life is a one-week retreat hosted by Be in Health at our campus in Thomaston, Georgia. It is designed to help people who are seeking healing and restoration of their physical, emotional, and spiritual health. We believe that most diseases result from separation in relationship from God, ourselves, and others. This retreat will help you to identify and deal with the "root issues" that may be keeping you from being in health. The For My Life retreat consists of intensive teachings, group ministry sessions, time to interact with the teachers and ask questions, and a time for personal prayer for healing at the end of the week.

Be in Health endeavors to make For My Life a safe place for you to find hope and healing for your life. We also offer For My Life Online for those who cannot travel at this time.

WALK OUT® WORKSHOP

After For My Life, the next step is the Walk Out Workshop (WOW). The term walk out refers to the journey of walking out of the old life of disease and hopelessness and entering into a new life of health and wholeness. During this one-week workshop, our team and attendees roll up their sleeves and begin to get really interactive with the principles from For My Life. We will talk about topics such as how to not go into guilt when we fall short, becoming established in our identity, overcoming temptation, how to forgive when you've been hurt, and learning to walk in the Father's love. Break-out groups, lots of Q & A, and continued healing of your spirit, soul, and body are all part of this amazing week.

FOR MY LIFE EXPANDED

This retreat will take you even deeper into the Be in Health teachings than For My Life and the Walk Out Workshop. You will receive a more thorough understanding of the specific spiritual roots of major disease classes. And will further uncover how the enemy works behind these diseases. This retreat will help you overcome diseases in your life and even help to prevent further diseases later. You will also participate in powerful corporate times of prayer and ministry after discussion times. For My Life Expanded is offered online for those who cannot travel at this time.

FOR MY LIFE® KIDS AND FOR MY LIFE® YOUTH

Every year in June and July, we offer For My Life for the whole family; that is the For My Life Adult, For My Life Youth (ages 13–17), and For My Life Kids' (ages 6–12) Retreat all in the same week! This is an opportunity for the whole family to be transformed and healed from the inside out. We hear so many people say, "If only I had known this when I was younger, I would have been saved from so much torment and heartache!" We've listened and developed these specialized retreats to continue our mission of establishing generations of overcomers. In the For My Life family week, everybody in the family can benefit and be on the same page spiritually. We take the same information that is presented in the adult For My Life Retreat, but reformat it to be relevant and engaging for each audience.

WOW KIDS

After the For My Life family weeks, we have the WOW family weeks. This is an opportunity for the whole family to come and learn how to be overcomers together. The WOW Kids class (ages 6–12) will equip your kids with the skills that they need to be overcomers. With a fun, engaging format, games, activities, and special "tools for freedom," your kids are sure to have a blast, make lasting memories, make new friends, and come out with valuable resources that will help them on their overcomer journey throughout their lives.

THE OVERCOMERS' COMMUNITY®

The journey of being an overcomer can be challenging, and we don't want you to have to do it alone. That is why we've developed the Overcomers' Community. This is a membership-based online forum dedicated to being a safe place for you to connect with the Be in Health team as well as with other overcomers. You can ask questions, get support and encouragement, share testimonies, find specific spiritual roots of diseases, have access to a wide selection of complete teachings and exclusive content, and more! We look forward to joining you in your walk-out journey and being able to assist you. With God's help, we can do this together! To learn more, go to: beinhealth.com/overcomers-community/.

BE IN HEALTH® CONFERENCES NEAR YOU

Our Be in Health team travels too! We bring one- to three-day conferences to locations all over the world. If you want to find out more about these conferences and when one might be held in your area, or if you are interested in helping us bring a conference to your area, go to: beinhealth.com.

SPIRITUAL LIFELINE®

Spiritual Lifeline is hands-on assistance and a ministry of love by the Be in Health team; it is our most individualized form of ministry to you. Our Father promises to deliver us from the enemy as we apply His Word. Together, we'll look at God's plan for your situation and His promises that will sustain you. This is all provided over the phone or through an online voice- or video-calling platform. Spiritual Lifeline is not a starting place at Be in Health, but is designed to come alongside and assist those who have previously attended our For My Life Retreat, or who have read and are applying the principles of Dr. Wright's books A More Excellent Way and Exposing the Spiritual Roots of Disease. Further information is available at: beinhealth.com/phone-ministry/

HOPE OF THE GENERATIONS CHURCH

Be in Health is a ministry of Hope of the Generations Church (HGC), a local body of believers located in Thomaston, Georgia. HGC is a nondenominational church and follows the model of the first-century church that was set in place by the apostles. We believe that every church, regardless of its background or diversity, should witness the same things recorded in the Bible: signs, wonders, healings, and miracles. These are life-altering tools of God to establish the authenticity of His Word. Join us Sunday mornings at 10:00 a.m. EST or Friday nights at 7:00 p.m. EST. We also stream our church services on our YouTube channel: youtube.com/c/BeinHealth.

A.C.T.S. GLOBAL; ASSOCIATION OF CHURCHES TEACHING AND SERVING®

Have you considered that God may be calling you to start, pastor, and establish a local church or gathering? Have the teachings of Be in Health opened your eyes, and now you want to tell others? Do you love people and want to see God's best for their life? Do you have a desire to guard the purity of the Bible and share that with others? Do you already, or do you desire to, gather people together to grow, heal, and fellowship together? Do people come to you for help and direction for their lives? Are you ready to be a pastor, but are held back by a lack of resources and training? If you answered yes to one or more of these questions, A.C.T.S. is here to help you take the next step. For more information, go to: actsglobal.com.

BE IN HEALTH® BLOG

The Be in Health Blog offers Biblical insights in a selection of articles about spiritual principles, overcoming, roots to diseases, and more. In addition, there are inspiring testimonies that are sure to encourage you in your own journey. It is updated weekly, so there is a continual flow of uplifting articles available for our readers. Find us at: beinhealth.com/blog/.

BE IN HEALTH® E-MAIL LIST

Do you want to stay connected with Be in Health and receive updates, messages from our pastors, news, events, and blog posts directly in your inbox? Then, sign up for Be in Health's mailing list at: beinhealth.com.

SOCIAL MEDIA

You can also follow us on your favorite social media platform!

Facebook: @beinhealth
Instagram: @hgc_bih
YouTube: @BeInHealth
Twitter: @BeinHealth

RESOURCES

Be in Health offers many other books and teachings from Dr. Wright, along with other members of the leadership team. All of the resources mentioned in this book are available on our website. Visit resources.beinhealth.com/ to find resources such as:

A More Excellent Way by Dr. Henry W. Wright
Exposing the Spiritual Roots of Disease by Dr. Henry W. Wright
7 Steps to Sin by Dr. Henry W. Wright
LORD God Revelation by Dr. Henry W. Wright Overcoming Allergies by Dr. Henry W. Wright
God is Greater Than Cardiovascular Disease by Dr. Henry W. Wright
Real Solutions for Autoimmune Disease by Pastors John and Adrienne Shales
Insights Into Cancer by Dr. Henry W. Wright
Overcoming Depression by Dr. Henry W. Wright Overcoming PTSD by Dr. Henry W. Wright
And much more!

About the Author

Dr. Henry W. Wright will be remembered for a great many things. His contributions to the health and welfare of the body of Christ were invaluable and continue to bear the wonderful fruit of healing and deliverance throughout the world. Yet to those who knew him, he was a genuine, sincere man who truly cared for each individual that he encountered.

He was fun-loving, with a sense of humor that could sometimes fly under the radar and other times catch you completely off guard. He deeply loved his wife, Pastor Donna Wright, his family, and his extended church family. And though he liked to keep the atmosphere light and encouraging, he took his role as a shepherd of the church very seriously.

It would be impossible to measure the impact he had on the lives of the people around him. His heart was to lead others to wholeness and peace in the love of God, and He did his best to represent God's love in all that he did. He would frequently say, "Healing is just a bonus. Our relationship with Father God, the Lord Jesus Christ, and the Holy Spirit is the most important thing that makes everything else work." He'd also say that he was just a guy doing what God told him to do. He didn't have to prove that he was something special; he wanted to lead others to God's love. Yet, because he yielded to God, God was able to use him mightily as a vessel for the furtherance of His Kingdom.

Dr. Wright was the president and founder of Hope of the Generations Church and Be in Health®. Together, Henry and Donna Wright faithfully taught and ministered to those that God sent to them. They also traveled all over the world, teaching conferences and ministering. Over time, God led them to establish the For My Life® Retreat and other subsequent retreats and conferences. These have led tens of thousands of people to restoration and healing in God as they learned the spiritual roots of disease and applied the scriptural truth to their lives.

Dr. Wright's first book, *A More Excellent Way*, was initially self-published, yet it became a bestseller on the Christian book marketplace, selling hundreds of thousands of copies worldwide. This book has helped thousands of people recover from the devastation of disease and find healing in God. *A More Excellent Way* is also translated into seven languages.

The book he published shortly before he went on to be with the Lord entitled, *Exposing the Spiritual Roots of Disease*, has already become an invaluable resource. He also left a wealth of insights and teachings that teach God's people how to walk as victorious overcomers in health and wholeness in every area of their lives—spirit, soul, and body.

Because of his extensive Biblical and medical research and understanding, he earned an honorary doctorate of therapeutic counseling from Chesapeake Bible College. He understood that we were more than just physical and psychological beings, we are also very spiritual after the image of God. That understanding was groundbreaking in helping people be recovered to wholeness in God in their whole being. He went on to develop the groundbreaking field of study called PneumaPsychoSomatology®, which studies the connection between the spirit, soul, and body according to the Bible.

His legacy will continue to bring healing and restoration to many more people. He put his hand to the plow and did not look back; he kept the faith and finished his course on the earth. Although we all greatly miss his presence with us, the day he went home to the Lord was the happiest day of his life. We rejoice with him on his graduation, and now it's our responsibility to continue submitting ourselves to God so that we too can be His vessels to complete the Lord's work here.

KING ST.

Set Three
BOOK 9

The Pub Trip

The Pub Trip
King Street: Readers Set Three - Book 9
Copyright © Iris Nunn 2014

Text: Iris Nunn
Editor: June Lewis

Published in 2014 by Gatehouse Media Limited

ISBN: 978-1-84231-134-9

British Library Cataloguing-in-Publication Data:
A catalogue record for this book is available from the British Library

One day Sid said to his wife, Brenda,
"You know,
things are looking up at the pub
now that we have live music.
I was thinking,
why don't we organise a pub outing?"

Brenda was quite surprised.
But then she thought a bit and said,
"Well, that's a lovely idea.
Where do we start?"

So, Sid went into town
to the travel agent's.

He said, "What sort of day trips
could you recommend?"

The travel agent said,
"There's Blackpool.
There's a trip to Amsterdam.
There's shopping in Birmingham.
There's a day trip to London.
And there are day trips to Ireland."

Sid took home lots of leaflets
and he and Brenda sat down
to look at them.

Later that evening he had a word
with Steve and Shane.

Together they thought about
the important things -

the cost,
the timing,
whether the trip would suit everyone

- and they voted for Ireland.

Steve made a poster on his computer.
It said:

PUB OUTING

Saturday 21st August
TO IRELAND

Leaving by coach from
The King's Arms
at 6.30am PROMPTLY

Returning to the pub at
2.30am on 22nd August

£25 per head

to include a packed lunch
(made by Brenda and Steve!)

All welcome - sorry no dogs

Well, there was a lot of talk
along the street about the outing.

Sam wanted to go,
but he was worried about Jim.

Jill wanted to go, but she said
she'd have to get the day off work.

Jane wanted to go, but she said
the twins might be sea-sick.

Steve put his name down
there and then.

Ros said she'd have to have a word
with Mrs T.

Sally said,
"I can help look after the children
on the boat."

June and Bob said,
"It'll be a great day out
for the whole family.
Let's take Grandad as well.
He'd enjoy the trip."

Mrs T said she'd like to go,
but she couldn't leave the shop.

Then Frank said
he'd look after the shop
and Mrs T said, "All right then.
Thanks Frank."

Sid and Brenda's children -
Jenny (and her son, Tony) and Pete -
said they would come too.

Mr and Mrs Javindra said
they would love to go to Ireland.

Bill and Ann said,
"It would be their second honeymoon!"

And that's how they filled
their 30 seater coach!